Health Transforming Foods | Their Stories and Recipes

KATHRYN BARI-PETRITIS

Library of Congress Control Number: 2021905354

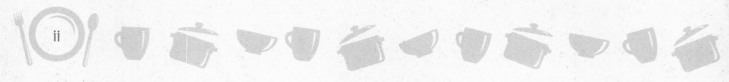

To my Mom, the late Judge Pearl B. Corrado, who inspired me to eat clean and simple and work hard.

To my Dad, the late Frank Corrado, for always believing in me.

To my husband Anthony, who has supported me on this journey in so many ways. His laughter energizes me.

To my son Christian, for always being my rock, for his dedication
and hard work at The Health Conscious Café.

To my daughter Melina, whose beautiful spirit inspires me daily.

To my grandsons Santino and Luca, who own a big piece of my heart.

Contents

Good morning, Breakfast! 58

Healthy Goodies 65

Educational Resources

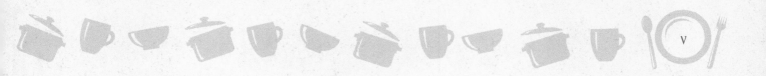

Forward

I was lucky enough to have the experience of working with my mother, and author of this special book, when we opened and ran The Health Conscious Chef Cafe during the late nineties in Long Island, New York. I cannot say enough how truly amazing it was to watch her shine by utilizing her innate talents as a cook, and her knowledge as a Whole Foods Chef during that time.

Before working with my mom at the café, I would describe her as kind, caring, nourishing, and loving. Incredibly, I watched my mom take this to another level as the chef and "Mother" to all the people that came into our shop. So many of those people needed that extra help with their diet, whether it be to help combat a specific ailment, or just to feel better and more alive everyday. Mom took the time with everyone to get to know them and recommend foods that would help. We knew almost all of them by name and they got such satisfaction from coming to a place where they could not only get a healthy meal, but could talk to the sweet woman behind the counter who offered a shoulder to lean on.

The menu and philosophy at The Health Conscious Chef was that of wholesomeness and education. Not only did mom utilize the skills and knowledge gleaned from being a graduate of The Natural Gourmet Institute (the Leader in Health Supportive Culinary Arts and Theory) to create a whole foods menu that was delicious and appealing to even "mainstream" diners, but she took on the task of teaching our customers why they should be eating these foods. I will never forget the poem she wrote about and called, "The Liver" in first person narration describes the importance of foods that help cleanse our bodies. While I laughed and made fun of this at the time as it hung in a fancy frame above our seating area, everybody read it and learned something. If they did not eat beets before, they strongly considered it at the liver's suggestion! It did not stop there, as each little sign for the dishes that sat in our display case had a note about the main ingredient, or a story attached. Quinoa grows on the highest mountains in subfreezing temperatures; surely it must be the strongest of the grains!

One of her cooking talents that made our shop so successful was her ability to transform a dish that in its original design was not meant to be healthy (only to taste good) and make it both delicious and health-supportive. Who would not want to order Eggplant Parmesan or Vegetable Lasagna? The eggplant slices were baked, not fried, with a soy cheese and an organic tomato sauce. The lasagna had five vegetables that were just lightly steamed with a homemade "ricotta" that you could swear was the real thing. These are just two examples (also foods from our Italian heritage that had been cooked and eaten for years in the traditional way) that allowed our store to appeal to the average eater. Of course right next to them on display was a Hijiki Seaweed Salad and a Teriyaki Tempeh Stir Fry. One might start with what they recognized but eventually they learned about and tried something new.

While we had a great run and eventually moved on from that location, Mom continued on as a private chef, teacher, and author. What remained consistent throughout were these qualities - transforming healthy foods, educating about them, and truly caring and nourishing those she taught and cooked for. I think you will see from the format of this book what it is I mean. I hope that when you cook these carefully thought out recipes that you will not only have a smile on your face with every bite and come away feeling nourished, but you will have a sense that you know why it was important you made them... and want to cook them for someone you love.

My sister and I had the wonderful experience of having a great chef for a mom. She always took the time every night to make us a home cooked meal. I was lucky enough to be a part of the progression of her education and the perfecting of her craft. Now I hope that you the reader will get to experience a little slice of what it means to be taken under Kathryn's wing.

Buon Appetito!
Christian Bari

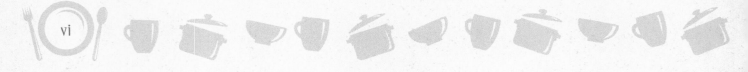

Introduction

We live in a time of revolutionary insights about health and nutrition. There are now hundreds of scientifically documented articles about the benefits of Real Food. Real Food has the power to transform your life.

What's Real Food? It's food that is genuinely fresh from the earth; organic when possible, grown as close to where you live as possible. It's simple, uncomplicated food that is easy to digest. These are nutrient dense foods, vibrant, heart healthy, full of oxygen, deep green cruciferous veggies and salad greens. It's food with a short shelf life.

My definition covers almost all fruits, vegetables in season, wheat grass, raw and sprouted seeds and nuts, seeds such as chia, hemp and flax. It includes the foods that are known for longevity; organic (when possible) whole grains, beans and legumes, fermented foods like sauerkraut, pickles, yogurt (low sugar ones), miso (from whole soybeans), butter, whole eggs, wild salmon and sardines. In my list, I also include free range, hormone-free animal products like chicken, turkey, bison, and lamb.

From my 20 years of experience as a holistic chef, I've seen that eating real, wholesome, and healthy food prepared with love and care can transform illness, create energy and vibrancy at any age, and cause people to say "You're HOW old?" very often.

Both your body and your brain improve when you commit to eating and cooking nourishing Real Foods. Today there is an emergence of a new consciousness about the impact of our food and our eating habits on our health. Cooking Real Foods is a learning experience that will expand your world in many ways. Cooking and sharing the foods in this book connects you to the hundreds of people that have enjoyed them before you and all the people who will start to enjoy them when you start serving them to friends and family.

Children who experience regular family meals with parents do better in every part of their lives – better grades, better health and better, healthier relationships. Regular meals at home with family help protect girls from developing eating issues like bulimia, anorexia, and from taking diet pills. Regular healthy meals reduce the incidence of childhood obesity as well.

Today we are actively examining why other cultures are living longer, healthier lives and experiencing less illness and disease. We learn that the answers include a positive outlook, an attitude of gratitude and a simple, wholesome diet of Real Food, usually prepared at home and shared with friends and family members. When older cultures maintain their native diet, their children are free from our American diseases. There is a powerful lesson here.

One hundred years ago we ate local organic food. We ate grass-fed animal products and whole food such as whole grains, legumes, beans and fermented food. Looking back in my Grandmother's day, most food was produced organically using farming methods that helped sustain the environment. There was no other way. There were no fast-food restaurants, no junk food, no frozen food, no packaged food to go, and no food bars. We ate what our mother or grandmother made for us. Most meals were eaten at home.

Sadly, we have lost that tradition and with it, the sacredness of a home cooked meal. As a nation, I believe we have lost sight of what constitutes Real Food and the powerful real connections we make when we prepare it and eat it together joyfully and gratefully.

My mission with this book is to turn you on to the idea that supercharging your life with the power of Real Foods and real connections will transform your health, your body and your relationships. The 25 recipes I have chosen for this book come from the list of "favorites" that my clients (and my family) have asked for over and over again in the last 20 years. Every recipe has a story. Some of the stories will tell you about nutrients and others will share experiences. All will bring a new dimension to your appreciation of the recipe and its ingredients.

Historically, the loving preparation of food is an activity that has the power to ground and center the family as they work together to make a meal happen (and then disappear). Activities like shared prepping and cooking make for a nice place to talk about the significant things that happened that day. It's why everyone gathers in the kitchen.

In my house, it's the place to be. No matter how many times I suggest my family and friends enjoy another area of the house, every time I turn around they are back in the kitchen. My kids grew up here and now that they are parents themselves, I see how much of a positive impact it made on them.

I recommend that you cook with soul in your kitchen. Be in the moment and give it your full attention. Be present with gratitude for your food and whatever state of health you are in. It's important to remember that good health is a journey. I'm happy you've begun it.

If you are a parent, now is the time to get involved when there is still an opportunity to be heard. Now is the time to buy and prepare fresh Real Food and bring it back to the family table. Stay away from packaged and processed foods. Parents are the gatekeepers of the family meals. Parents need now, more than ever, to implement healthier food choices. I agree with the wise words of Dr. Brian Clement PH.D. and Co-Director of the Hippocrates Institute, "Health will not happen tomorrow unless we intentionally create it today."

As a health conscious mother and grandmother, I live by those words. As a teacher of holistic health I make sure my clients have that sentiment in front of them every day. I ask them to think about the journey of healthy cooking and eating like they are training for a sport – set some goals, get some feedback and make adjustments along the way.

It's time to think about making new choices when it comes to food. Today, I'm concerned about the supply of good, wholesome, chemical-free and drug-free food. My choices reflect that.

Now is the time to justify purchasing and eating organic foods, which include clean, hormone and antibiotic-free animal products. It's time to say "NO" to genetically modified products and demand proper labeling of those foods so you know what you are putting into your mouth and the mouths of your family. Genetically Modified Organisms (GMO'S) are created by altering DNA. I'm not interested in feeding dangerous food to my family. Start your own research on the topic, and you'll likely agree with me.

Refuse to bring into your house trans fats, high fructose corn syrup (now labeled corn solids), white sugar, salt that is not mineral rich (as some sea salts are) and industrialized, processed foods. Eliminate soy protein (even

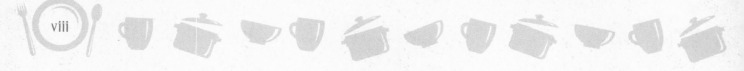

"natural" soy protein). Soy protein can be bathed in a toxic, explosive chemical solvent known as Hexane.[1] 94% of soy is GMO.[2]

You need to pay attention to the soy protein that can be found in thousands of vegetarian products such as: prepackaged veggie burgers; veggie cheese; bakery items, tuna fish in cans, protein drinks and bars, and most alarmingly, in infant formula products. Hexane is a petroleum chemical produced as a by-product of gasoline refining. It is used to process nearly all conventional soy protein ingredients but is prohibited when processing organic foods.[3]

Be vigilant and practice defensive shopping by reading labels and understanding the ingredients on your favorite boxed or canned foods, if you're still buying them.

I teach many young parents. In their efforts to find healthy eating options, they are eager to learn about the hidden names for MSG so they won't be tricked into buying it. See the great list we put together for you in the back of this book along with other hidden names for additives, preservatives and fillers on packaged foods. Become a detective, it's kind of fun. I've developed an "eagle eye" over time and can find the hidden sugar, sodium, GMO'S, MSG and artificial ingredients on almost all labels. Does that mean I never buy them? No. It means I make informed choices.[4]

In parts of Europe and in Australia, most artificially colored foods have to carry the warning: "may have an adverse effect on activity and attention in children." Parents underestimate how many additives their children actually eat. The good news is that you can join support groups with other parents and help each other collect relevant information and then act upon it. You can refuse to support products and companies that endanger your health; you can make informed choices and still eat wholesome and delicious food.

Let my story be the catalyst for change in your life. Let the stories of the food and the recipes that have been beloved by the people I've been blessed to cook for expand your world, enchant and surprisingly delight your palate.

"My Story" by Chef Kathryn Bari-Petritis

Writing this book has been on my "bucket list" for years now, but life happened, and I put it on the back burner. As I celebrate my twentieth year of professional healthy cooking with passion, I've chosen to honor clients, my work and myself by putting this very special book out to the world. What you read here is how I live my life everyday - with mindful, conscious eating.

I believe we all deserve wellness for a lifetime. My deepest hope is that my book and my story will spark that intention within you, and from your intention will come the passion to change your life, and the lives of those you love, for the better.

When I was 19, my Mom developed an interest in the work of nutritionist Adele Davis and shared with me what she was learning. She started taking Vitamin C and invested in some quality supplements. *A window to new thinking about food and health opened up for me.*

At 31, after a sad divorce, with two young children, I really needed to make life-altering changes. As a single mother thrown into the work force I found I needed two things to juggle it all - good real food and exercise. *If I was to take stellar care of those kids I needed to be strong and stay healthy.*

I read everything there was to read at the time on Macrobiotics and whole food cooking. I started with hearty lentil and chickpea soups, and spinach and broccoli pies. I made sure we had family meals together every night. I often had to make up fun songs about broccoli being brain food to capture the children's attention, but it worked. To this day they still remember that they ate their green veggies, in part due to my songs.

We made mealtimes fun but there was no negotiating on food choices like I witness today with young families. I worked hard to buy and prepare the food and the children came to respect that.

My meals then were part of what's now known as a "Rainbow Diet." All the colors represent foods rich in anti-oxidants, with lots of phytochemicals. We didn't realize then how vital these colors would be to our long-term health.

The year 1990 was a turning point in my life. I started to see much sickness around me. A dear friend of mine died of cancer and my twin brother developed MS. That was both sad and scary for me.

By the time I hit 40 the next year, my diet had evolved into something greater. I studied a lot of Gary Null's books on nutrition and learned to figure out my own biochemistry. I came to understand which foods really gave me optimum energy and vitality. Learning my blood type (O-Positive) and applying the right foods for that type helped me feel even better.

One day while running on my treadmill at home, I had an enlightening experience. The Japanese Buddhists call it "satori." It means "awakening."

At that very moment it became crystal clear to me that I was called to help people make better food choices by teaching what simple, uncomplicated, healthy Real Food is.

I was on my true path to learn more.

After researching a few schools in New York, I enrolled in "The Natural Gourmet Institute for Food and Health" in New York City. They are truly "the leader in health-supportive culinary arts and theory." It's a *one of a kind, culinary school*, integrating body, mind and spirit in its teaching philosophies.

After I graduated, I started a home business cooking for a select group of people. I turned my dining room into a commercial kitchen and started collecting huge pots, bowls and containers that held pounds of healthier foods. I filled storage bins with organic grains and beans and so started my journey to provide the world with better food and lifestyle choices.

I designed a weekly menu consisting of a wide variety of delicious seasonal foods and healthier desserts. I took orders joyfully and soon had a loyal following showing up at my door on Mondays and Fridays for their pick-ups.

In 1995, my son Christian Bari, a business major, graduated from Boston University and returned home. He started helping me with computer work and organizing what was soon to be called "The Health Conscious

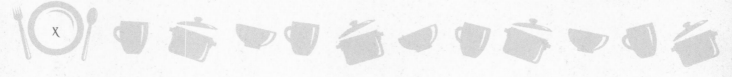

Chef." I was still operating out of my house but soon needed to find real space to serve customers in a more professional way.

My sister JoAnna, a business owner and author, created a tag line for the business, which graces my business cards to this day, it reads, "Wholesome Foods to Support your Healthier Lifestyle." My daughter Melina, a savvy businesswoman, contributed her bright ideas about marketing and advertising.

My Mom, Pearl Corrado, a retired Supreme Court Justice helped us financially and took a strong interest in the business. So, in 1997, the three of us, three generations, Mom, Christian and I began a journey together opening up shop.

We found what we thought was a wonderful location in an unused hotel kitchen and we gave it our all. We started out as a healthy take-out spot, but soon customers wanted to stay and have their eating experience there. Since we didn't advocate "eating on the run," my dad and I ran around town finding second hand tables and chairs and charming, soulful, crafty kitchen décor. We decorated the place in a pinch of time. I sewed some curtains and shopped some antique stores for various eclectic kitchen accessories from the 50's and 60's. It all worked; people loved it. "The Health Conscious Chef" now resembled a cozy, colorful café straight out of Greenwich Village or Soho, New York City. We provided people with energizing organic foods, meals, desserts and snacks. We had a raw juice bar, wheatgrass shots, and a retail section of natural foods and key supplements.

We had a few wholesale accounts too. Owners of other health foods stores, deli's and even a gym now sold our special foods. Our Rainbow Turkey Veggie Loaf was a big hit with the weight lifters – it tasted great and was power-packed with protein. A year into the business I was approached by the owner of several Jewish Delis. He wanted some lighter, healthy additions to his menu. It was a great opportunity for us and so we did all that was necessary to become Kosher.

Sadly, like many small family businesses, we were forced to close after a few short years. The café was never zoned for sit down eating (only take-out.)

We were forced to look at every aspect of the business to help us make that expensive decision. When we looked at it with a critical eye, we had to face the factors that were not in our favor as well as the ones that were. We didn't own the property, we were located down a side street with no traffic light, and we were in the basement of a hotel kitchen. The only way people could see us from the street at all was a life-size wooden statue of me wearing a large white chef's hat and smiling while displaying the daily specials. What they say about "Location, location, location" is true. The location didn't really support the business well and it didn't make financial sense to invest more money and time in it.

It was pretty devastating, especially because we were disappointing our loyal customers. They were calling us for the longest time not knowing why we closed such a "wonderful happy place." Rents had become just too high for us in that area on the north shore of Long Island; our customers were *there* and our homes were there. It didn't make sense to move away and start all over again.

I look back in gratitude for all of it. I feel blessed to have served the community as best I could for as long as I did. There was precious time spent with family, friends and new acquaintances. You can't put a price tag on that.

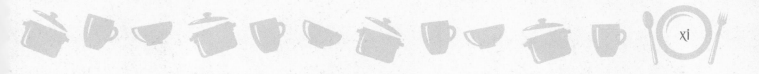

When the store closed, I chose not to dwell on the negative so I started to do private cooking for a few customers. My son got a job in Manhattan and adjusted well to the change. I taught my children never to fear the unknown – and that one job may be a giant stepping stone to something better. Today, my son enjoys his work in the real estate market in New York City and Brooklyn and maintains a healthy lifestyle with his lovely wife and baby boy.

While I was building my private cooking business, a few new opportunities appeared. I presented many seminars and lectures on a variety of important topics in health and nutrition. For years I was involved in producing educational demos and lectures at Stony Brook University on Long Island. That inspired many young students to examine and change their poor diets. To this day I still hear from a few of them. Those lectures profoundly changed their lives.

I had a creative and informative website designed by my nephew Mark, which definitely helped to build awareness of my new business. Today I am constantly adding new material to that original website. TheHealthChef.com gets more colorful and more useful each year.

In 2001 some very special people appeared in my life, and in my opinion, not by chance. Kathleen McBride and Carol Gevisenheit were both lovely sweet women. Both were young, talented and had beautiful children and adoring husbands. Both lost their battles with cancer and left such a huge void behind.

My cooking and caring for them reassured me that my work as a Health Chef was divinely guided. Their strength and devotion to healthy eating was a huge inspiration to me. They were my teachers and I will forever carry them in my heart. They changed my life forever.

Eight years later I was introduced to Tracy and Paul Posillico. At the age of five weeks, their precious baby girl Whitney was diagnosed with a malignant Rhabdoid tumor of the kidney. The doctors gave her parents the devastating report that she had a 20% chance of survival. The family asked me to join their team, which they called "Team Whitney", and I did so joyfully. Tracy was nursing Whitney on demand around the clock and needed to keep her daily calorie intake at around 3200 to keep her breast milk robust.

She needed the purest, freshest foods I could find, in other words, the Real Food I spoke about in the introduction to this book. Her breast milk was an important, vital, necessary factor in Whitney's recovering weekly from some of the strongest chemotherapy treatments known. The doctors didn't believe that a child this small would make it through the treatment so successfully, but she did. The staff at Sloane Kettering Hospital nicknamed her "the rockstar." A special friend and colleague, Chef Jill Engelhart joined "Team Whitney" and worked with me weekly creating nutrient-dense meals for Tracy, Whitney and Paul.

Chef Jill and I love to remind each other now how Whitney enjoyed so many different ethnic foods, like cauliflower chickpea curry stew. When she sat in her high chair she would stare out at all shapes and colors as we were washing all the produce. She knew what good foods were about to come! She always ate with gusto and joy.

Whitney lived two weeks past her first birthday. Tracy's parents and I spoke afterwards on how much we admired Tracy's commitment to eating pure, fresh and whole foods every day. She drank up to three greens juices a day to nourish her through nursing. Tracy never missed a beat every day, taking all her foods back

and forth to the hospital when Whitney was there. She definitely added months to Whitney's life even after so many professionals gave her so little hope.

What exquisite love was demonstrated by these two parents! Whitney lives on through the money raised for the research of pediatric cancer. If you want to make a difference in the research see the footnote below.[6]

I love working with people who are healthy and want to get healthier. I love working with families who want to blueprint their kids with good habits from the start. I recognize though, that the most rewarding aspects of my career have been working with families who endured enormous sadness. For me, these transforming experiences are lessons that cannot be learned in a classroom.

We can hope that someday soon there will be cures for so many of the terrible diseases that plague our nation now and we can take action to do our best to prevent them. Learn what you can from this book and then spread the word to friends, family and co-workers who are eating dead, empty calories and frequenting establishments that use cheap oils, and toxic products in their cooking. If their prices are cheap, chances are that is the case. You can find healthier and organic items in even some of the largest superstores today. Do your homework before shopping!

I want to inspire you to expand your awareness of the pleasure of cooking for yourself and those you love dearly. I ask you to eat consciously with appreciation and gratitude and watch what happens! Choose foods that bring balance and nourishment to you, supporting body, mind and spirit. At the same time, you will be supporting the health of your environment and on a much larger scale, the health of the earth.

The most important thing I learned in school is that complete nourishment is made up of *more* than the macronutrients, calories, vitamins and minerals found in the food itself. An old Chinese proverb says that it is truly the "Chi of the Chef" – *the life force energy of the Cook* - that permeates the food. It's not so much the skills in the kitchen that you have but the creative force, love and passion for delicious food that will make you a good cook. When shopping, chopping, preparing and eating is done with reverence and love you elevate and transform the activity into a blessed experience.

Now you know my story. It's time to take a look at yours. Are you ready to intentionally create more health and wellness in your life?

Here's what you need to put this easily adaptable plan into action:

Commit to learning something new every day. (Even professional chefs do this - they may be improving or creating new meals.) Trying a new recipe is a great exercise for your brain. There is so much amazing information out there now on brain health. The brain is a muscle that must be used and challenged. *Experts are saying to do a crossword puzzle, and I say challenge yourself with one of my recipes that you haven't tried before.*

And now as you begin to construct a nutrient-dense diet:

* Build your immunity and stamina with confidence by honoring yourself and lovingly feed your body.
* Engage the energy of cooking with joy; shift your consciousness on learning about and eating new foods. Say, "I can do this; it's a new adventure that I will embrace today."

* Expand your horizons with a diverse diet. Choose a wide variety of colorful foods and rotate your foods every day, especially proteins. Be aggressive with a new approach to dark leafy greens. Chop them, juice them, sauté them with spices for bold flavors, bake them in casseroles and stews and even eat them in the morning with eggs in a burrito!

* Shop for wholeness. In doing so, you're shopping for health and healing. Have fun navigating through the beautiful and interesting markets around your town. Visit your local outside markets when weather permits. Look up at the blue sky and feel the blazing sun and buy sun-ripened local produce, even if it is not organic. "Freshly picked" still has special nutrients from the sun and the air. Stay alert and aware about avoiding GMO crops even at your local farm stand. There are eight crops for GM seeds that are commercially available in the US: corn, soybeans, canola, alfalfa, sugar beets, cotton, papaya and squash.

* Support your local farms, look into a CSA, (Community Supported Agriculture) near you. If possible, choose not to support mass-produced food and fast food.

* Stay away from GMO's.[4] Choose organic to be guaranteed by organic standards that no genetic modification has taken place in your foods. The newest developments in this technology are "pharm crops" - pharmaceutical drugs and vaccines grown on food (corn is one of the most common host plants.) The Organic Consumers Association and the Environmental Working Group offer lists of the most important foods to buy organic. Learn the list of the <u>"Dirty dozen" and "Clean 15"</u> fruits and vegetables.[5] Cleaner food translates to better health.

My friends, as you begin your journey reading, learning and trying my recipes, I suggest that you take these steps:

- Read each recipe thoroughly before starting to cook.
- Don't be intimated by any recipe; embrace it as a brain exercise and you will be smarter for it.
- Take note as to what can be prepared in advance, particularly for longer recipes.
- If it works for you, take a recipe and break it down into smaller components by using different colored sticky notes.
- Trust your instincts and creative energy throughout the cooking process.
- Taste and re-taste the dish after 20 minutes to make sure you are achieving the right flavors and textures.
- Be patient with yourself. There is a lot of trial and error involved; this is part of the improvisation in the kitchen. I really believe it's all about the practice. Practice at any trade will make you good.
- Invite a dear friend over to share the cooking experience and laugh a lot! Who says healthy cooking has to be hard?

Join me and let's get on the healthy cooking journey together – stress free - and cook wholeheartedly, abundantly and with joy and love.

God bless you richly.

Chef Kathryn
The Health Conscious Chef

"Our bodies are our gardens, to the which our wills are gardeners" ......Shakespeare

Soups, a Bowl of Comfort

When you are making healthy food choices, choose soup first. There are so many valuable nutrients in a soup. The vibrancy attracts us and the warmth of the soup sustains us. Personally, soup nourishes me on all levels; body, mind and spirit. Even when I was not a trained chef, making soup was a meaningful and soulful experience for me. Just stirring the soup, nursing the pot and thinking about those who would share the meal with me made the kitchen work pleasurable.

The criteria for planning soups is very much seasonal. In the beginning of fall and extending until January/February, all the orange and green speckled colored squashes are ripe. Here are some examples: Butternut, Kabocha, Turban, Sugar Pumpkin, Cheese Pumpkin, and Delicata. Pumpkins and squashes all belong to the same genetic family, however pumpkins are considered a fruit because it contains seeds.

This is the time of year to make a creamy butternut soup, which is a magnificent and universally loved soup. If you saw a butternut squash in your grocery store or local market in the summer, chances are it was grown very far from your home. There is a distinct natural sweetness in that squash, reminiscent of sweet potatoes, and cooking it in summer might lack in that sweet flavor making the soup somewhat flat. As we approach winter, all the root vegetables are in season and nothing can compare to the taste of a pureed squash or root soup, garnished with a cashew cream or yogurt swirl.

Soup must be in harmony with the whole menu. Some soups like Miso with ginger served before the main course can stimulate the appetite. Power-packed green soups can detox and energize at the same time. A variety of bean and grain soups can be super hearty for winter's months yet a creamy black soup with fresh corn and tomatoes and garnished with toasted tortillas on top can be a great summer soup.

In other countries they enjoy soups for breakfast. I often have a creamy soup for breakfast like my green split pea soup with wild rice, or a red lentil sweet potato soup. But heating them to a boil is not necessary, just enjoy slightly warmed to start your day with this bowl of pure bliss.

There are broth-based soups, bean soups, vegetable soups, cream soups, fruit soups and other types of soups. Soups are so versatile and have many uses. Some of the pureed thick soups are excellent over oatmeal or brown rice. Heartier vegetable or bean soups can be used as a base for casseroles, stews and other recipes. Soups have such different characters and are an ideal way to experience flavors from all over the world, making use of herbs and spices that distinguish national cuisines. Most soups will freeze well up to 3-4 months. I suggest if you defrost a soup for dinner or lunch, have a fresh colorful raw salad alongside the soup, since freezing soup will kill some vitamins and minerals on a cellular level.

I truly encourage you to make soups on a weekly basis. With wholesome organic ingredients they provide nourishing, easily assimilated food for young and old. Soup is a perfect way to get veggies into members of the family who normally say no to vegetables.

Nothing is as satisfying as a bowl of good soup, the ultimate comfort food. My mother's last meal was a creamy butternut soup that I made with so much love for her, one evening after work. Pleasure showed on her face when she sipped it. It was hard for her to digest food at that point, but this soup was ultimately satisfying to her and you can't put a price on that.

A Luscious Lima Bean Soup

This is a soup of mine that became everyone's favorite and goes back 15 years ago to *The Health Conscious Chef Café*.

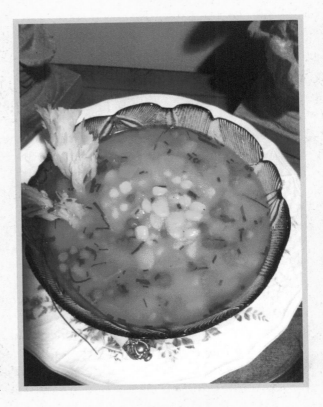

Customers have told me that the Lima Bean Soup is a rich tasting soup but without the calories to match. I promise you that you will not need to reach for a slice of bread or even crackers with this soup, it's that satisfying and full bodied. It has a warming effect on a cold night yet delightfully dazzling on a warm summer day, served room temp, topped with colorful ripe heirloom tomatoes and just picked fresh herbs from the garden. Give it a garnish blast of chopped red and orange peppers to delight the senses with summery flavors.

My little grandson has enjoyed this soup since he was 6 months, for him I pureed most of it. Now he can digest it whole, and still loves it but always with a kiss of parmesan cheese and a kiss from his Nanny.

The baby lima bean is less starchy than most other beans. It is highly *alkalizing* which is essential to our proper acid/alkaline balance, our pH level. It's sad to say that our American diet is an acid producing diet. The body must deal with acid on a regular basis, and our daily stress makes acid.

The body is an alkaline entity by design; strong acid in the body can damage tissue and cause pain. Eat 80% alkaline foods and 20% acid foods for perfect pH balance. Staying on an exercise program and eating close to Mother Nature is a good plan. In my opinion, the lima bean is one of the best beans for most Americans because it is an easy bean to digest (my recipe calls for soaking which aids in that). The bean is extremely versatile, and can be used in many health supportive dishes.

The baby lima beans are in a separate botanical classification than the large lima bean. Its texture is more buttery, a thinner skin. Both are called "The New World Beans." They are native to Peru, with origins that can be traced back to about A.D.1500 and christened lima after the capital of Peru. This bean is the favorite to the Native American who cooked it with a combination of fresh corn. This then became the popular Colonial dish mispronounced as "Succotash" from the Native American word *msickquatash*.

It's a simple soup to make and can really impress your family and company.

Luscious Lima Bean Soup

Yield: 8 servings

Ingredients:

1½ cups dry baby lima beans, washed, sorted and
    soaked 4-8 hours
9 cups water
¼ inch piece of Kombu seaweed, rinsed
1 tablespoon olive oil
1 medium onion, small dice
3 celery stalks, medium dice
3 carrots, medium dice

Optional:
1 large sweet potato, medium chop
1 butternut squash (when in season), medium chop

1 parsnip, medium chop
1½ teaspoons ground coriander
2 teaspoons sea salt, divided
¼ teaspoon freshly ground black pepper
1 teaspoon unsalted organic butter (optional)
1 cup fresh or frozen organic sweet corn, thaw if frozen
1 cup fresh or frozen petite organic green peas, thaw
    if frozen

Garnish:
¼ cup sliced scallions or chopped fresh chives

Procedure:

1. To create a creamy texture to beans, soak in 6 cups of water overnight. For a quick soak: add hot water to beans and soak for 4 hours. Drain and rinse. Discard soaking water.
2. In a 6-9 quart saucepan, bring 9 cups of water to a rolling boil. Add drained beans and Kombu. Return water to a boil and skim off foam. Cook 40-45 minutes. Beans should be soft, not mushy.
3. In a medium size frying pan or saucepan, sauté onion in olive oil until golden. Add coriander and stir to incorporate.
4. Add, celery, carrots, parsnip and butter, if using, one teaspoon salt, 1 cup water and bring to a boil. Cover, reduce heat to medium, and steam for 10 minutes.
5. Add the steamed veggies to soup pot. If soup is too thick, add ½ cup water.
6. Add remaining teaspoon of salt plus the pepper and simmer another ten minutes to blend flavors. Taste and adjust seasonings.
7. Remove from heat. Cool slightly before next step.
8. Ladle half the amount of soup into blender. Liquefy for 1 minute.
9. Separately steam the sweet potato and butternut squash, if using. Add to soup at the end so soup remains creamy white.
10. Return to pot. Add corn and peas. Adjust salt and pepper.
11. Garnish with scallions or chives.

Cook's Notes:

*   Try not to add additional water in order to keep the chowder-like consistency.
*   This is a thick soup that freezes well.
*   Peas and corn should be fresh, when possible.
*   When in season, adding one cup chopped cooked butternut squash gives a lovely flavor.
*   Check the "Bean Buzz" section of the book to read more about cooking beans from scratch and the benefits of using Kombu seaweed.

Southwestern Tomato and Vegetable Soup

This hardy colorful soup stars the black-eye pea along with the great crucifer collard greens. It's a soup that's loaded with vitamins and minerals and best of all, the taste is universal. "Mother Earth in her fullness."

When fresh local corn and ripe sun-kissed tomatoes are in season, the flavor screams at you, but organic frozen corn and some jarred plum tomatoes will capture the taste too.

In the South the black-eye pea is eaten on New Years Eve, to bring in good luck for the coming year. Collard greens are the number one dark green vegetable as rated on the ANDI Score (Aggregate Nutrient Density Index), for nutrient content. Here the cellular nutrition is all in one package. The sweetness of the corn, red pepper and tomatoes swirling around color and texture soothes any palette.

The soup has a special story in my family. My twin brother and sister, while traveling to New York in the winter of 2012, found themselves in some uncomfortable situations. My mom was critically ill in the hospital, and they stayed long hours and were fatigued. They both stayed at her place, but neither had energy to shop or cook and, when you're in that situation, going to restaurants is not where you want to be. I made a giant pot of this soup, and the story goes that they lived on it for three days. What ever was left, my brother brought back home with him, 6 hours away in West Chazy, New York. (In a cooler bag I packed for him, along with a hearty split pea soup I made). He added his own brown rice to the southwestern soup to extend its life for one more day. My twin brother and his wife now make this soup regularly.

I have also served this soup for big crowds at my home. My husband's family reunion was one of them. Along with some traditional Italian recipes I was serving, I was surprised how well it blended in and complimented the other dishes. I set up a big white crock pot of this soup, and kept it at a simmering temperature, next to a funky red and white enamel ladle from the forties. And of course, some great crusty country bread.

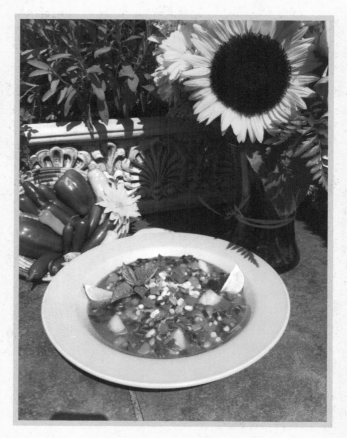

It just looks dreamy in the pot. Everyone enjoyed it so much. I even left copies of the recipes for everyone at the door when they were leaving. They really appreciated it. Soups like this one are the cornerstones of a heart-healthy stress free diet and also memories can be made with this soup. A fragrant simmering soup pot means love and simply joy.

Southwestern Tomato and Vegetable Soup

Yield: 8 servings

Ingredients:

1 cup dried black-eyed peas
1 bay leaf
¼ inch piece of Kombu seaweed, rinsed
1 tablespoon olive oil
1 medium Spanish onion, medium chop
1 small red onion, small chop
4 garlic cloves, minced
1 teaspoon ground coriander

½ teaspoon chili powder
1 teaspoon thyme
¼ teaspoon cayenne pepper
1 small jalapeno pepper, small chop
2 celery stalks, medium chop
4 small red potatoes, medium cubed
1 (22 ounce) can diced tomatoes, plus two cups water
2 teaspoons Tamari (wheat-free soy sauce)

1 cup (3 ounces) of collard greens, de-stemmed, cut into ¼-inch squares
1 cup fresh or frozen organic corn kernels
1 large red pepper, small chop
3 tablespoons chopped cilantro
2 teaspoons sea salt, divided
Freshly ground pepper to taste

Garnish:

4 scallions, white and greens parts, chopped

Optional garnish:

4 plum tomatoes, deseeded, medium dice

Procedure:

1. Combine the black-eyed peas, bay leaf, and Kombu in a medium size saucepan. Add enough water to cover the beans by 2 inches (about 7 cups water). Bring water to a boil over high heat. Stir frequently, adding more water if level gets too low. Cook 25 minutes, or until peas are soft, but still hold their shape.
2. Stir in 1 teaspoon salt, cook for 1 minute. Drain peas, saving 1 cup of cooking liquid to the side.
3. In a large soup pot, sauté the onions in olive oil until golden.
4. Add garlic, stir for 1 minute.
5. Add spices (except cayenne), jalapeno pepper and celery. Cook 5 minutes.
6. Add red potatoes and 6 cups of cold water. Bring to a boil and cook for 10 minutes.
7. Lower the heat, add the diced tomatoes and 2 cups water, and cook on low boil for ten minutes.
8. Add the Tamari, remaining teaspoon of salt, and ground pepper to taste.
9. Stir in collard greens and cayenne pepper. Cook for 5 minutes, stirring frequently. Continue on low heat.
10. Add the drained black eye peas with reserved cup of cooking liquid to pot and cook until greens are tender, stirring frequently (about 6 minutes).
11. Add corn, red pepper and cilantro. Stir well to blend. Adjust salt and pepper.
12. Add garnish and serve immediately.

Cook's Notes:

- You can chiffonade the collards. To chiffonade, first de-stem a piece of the leaf, roll up tight like a cigar, and slice through. It will taste the same but may be easier to chew.
- This recipe makes 12 cups. As I told the story in my forward, it is a great party soup served with corn chips, hummus, avocado and a splash of lime.
- Tamari is a wheat-free soy sauce. Please see *Japanese and Chinese Pantry* section in the back of the book.
- I suggest keep vegetable stock on hand. This soup may get thicker the following day. You can use 1-2 cups of stock to thin out during the reheating process.

Summertime and the living is easy with this Gazpacho Soup

Gazpacho is a classic summer beauty. It's a vibrantly colorful, chunky soup that is deeply nourishing too. It's an interesting play of spices. You can create a sweeter soup with fresh carrot juice versus tomato juice or go for a real kick with a pinch more cayenne pepper, and more chopped jalapeno pepper.

Apple cider vinegar is my choice of vinegar here. It's a combination of tart good taste and germ-killing acids. Apple cider vinegar contains more than thirty important nutrients, a dozen minerals, over half a dozen vitamins and essential acids, and several enzymes. Plus, it has a large dose of pectin for a healthy heart. While trying a host of different vinegars in this recipe, this one fit the puzzle.

I often start my day with a good friend and a drink of this amazing soup (at room temp.) It's refreshing and energizing because it is all raw.

The sad news is that you can not get the quality of tomatoes we need for this exceptional depth in taste in the winter months. That's why this is my Summer Gazpacho soup for the region in which we live. However if your home is in the warmer states, enjoy creating this soup anytime.

For the best of summer entertaining serve soup in small brandy glasses or other small glasses. Serve on a beautiful platter with nasturtium flowers and leaves. With the current popularity of all the heirloom tomatoes, use them for special garnish with delicate pieces of cilantro or basil. It makes a real statement about FRESH. Small is really the "big" here, it's trendy now to achieve this look for appetizers.

I served this soup at my daughter's garden bridal shower on a 92 degree day, a few summers ago on my patio. The ladies said it took the edge off the heat a bit. They loved the look of it also. You'll find many versions of this recipe all over the world; but mine is tried and true. Enjoy it, be cool.

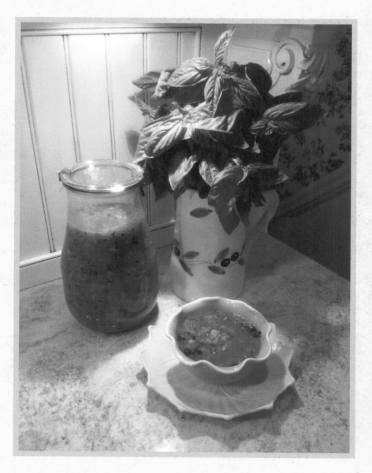

Summer Gazpacho Soup

Yield: 6 (1 cup) servings or 20 demi shot glasses

Ingredients:

8 ripe Italian plum tomatoes

4 vine-ripened tomatoes or 3 ripe beefsteak
tomatoes

2 large or 3 medium cucumbers (peel if not organic),
halved and deseeded

1 medium red bell pepper, cored and deseeded

2-inch cube green bell pepper

1 small red onion

3 garlic cloves, peeled

1 small jalapeno pepper

¼ cup Italian flat-leaf parsley, de-stemmed

¼ cup cilantro, de-stemmed

2 ½-3 cups tomato juice

2-3 tablespoons of apple cider vinegar

Sea salt and freshly ground pepper, to taste

Optional:
2 tablespoons olive oil

Garnish:
2 scallions (white and green parts), chopped

1 tablespoon fresh basil, chopped

1 yellow pepper, small dice

Procedure:

1. Wash all veggies in a vegetable wash.
2. Fast chop the tomatoes, cucumbers, bell peppers, red onion, and jalapeno.
3. In a high-quality blender or food processor, starting with the tomatoes and cucumbers, pulse vegetables and herbs in small batches (2 cups at a time).
4. While blender is on, alternate adding ingredients while slowly incorporating the tomato juice, making sure to adjust amount as not to make the soup too watery. You are looking to create a semi-chunky consistency, which makes it interesting.
5. Pulse in olive oil, if using.
6. Place contents into large bowl and adjust salt, pepper, and vinegar.
7. Chill for at least 1 hour. Top with garnishes just before serving.

Cook's Notes:

- Purchase tomato juice in glass jars.
- Soup will stay fresh for up to 5 days because of the vinegar.
- Note on this vinegar: Vinegar is credited with saving the lives of thousands of soldiers during the U.S. Civil War. It was routinely used as a disinfectant on wounds.

Bouillabaisse for every Season

Bouillabaisse is one of the most famous of all Mediterranean fish soups. Inspired by sunny days in Provence, it is a rich colorful mixture of fish and shellfish flavored with saffron, fennel, tomatoes and orange. I have added parsnip and potatoes to make it more of a one pot meal.

The fragrant and desirable spice used in this soup, is saffron. Saffron threads are the whole dried stigmas from the beautiful violet colored autumn crocus. About 75,000 flowers are needed to produce only one pound of saffron, which is why saffron is the world's most expensive spice. It is a necessary spice to create this festive dish, however you need only a very small amount of the threads. I love reading about the long history of this spice dating back to ancient times when different geographic regions developed their own culinary traditions using saffron to season a wide variety of dishes. Its deep rich layers of flavor and dazzling yellow-orange hues have an ethnic flair that you can recreate. It's worth putting the time and energy into creating this soup.

The aromatic smell of the saffron threads soaking in water, waiting to be mixed into the soup gets your excitement going, just knowing something wonderful is about to happen when that spice explodes into its flavor. Assembling the prep is key here, everything after that is pure joy.

Choose the freshest fish from your local fish market. Choosing good looking leeks, fennel and parsnip is a challenge in some markets, take time to choose the freshest. When you get home, kick off your shoes, open all windows like you might do in Provence, turn up the music and feel love for those whom will enjoy your masterpiece. For those who cannot eat shellfish it is perfectly fine to omit and substitute another fish.

Why not delight your whole family with this soup? It's a great weekend soup, because sometimes week days may be too hectic to put it all together. Do your homework and plan it out. No worries. There are health benefits galore in this delicious soup. Fish is a heart healthy food.

A favorite client of mine serves this soup a few times in the summer to special friends with just a great crunchy green salad and sweet citrus dressing to complement the soup. She says it's all they need for an exciting summer feast. Fresh snipped green herbs at the end are a sweet finale. This soup is also part of my love list of favorite meals for friends. Saffron makes for interesting conversation too, it's a known aphrodisiac.

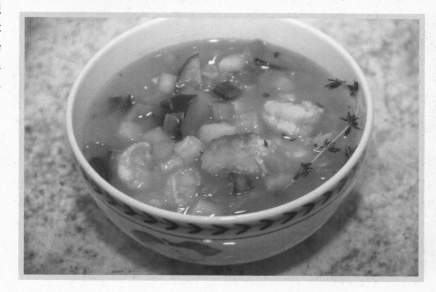

Bon Appétit!

Bouillabaisse for Every Season

Yield: 6-8 servings

Ingredients:

2 pounds fresh fish: halibut, dry scallops, cod or shrimp (shelled, deveined, and tails removed)

1 small Spanish onion, medium chop

6 garlic cloves, minced

1 leek, white part only, thinly sliced

1 golden potato, peeled, small chop

2 carrots, medium chop

3 celery stalks, medium chop

½ fennel bulb, small chop

1 medium parsnip, medium chop

½ teaspoon saffron threads plus 2 tablespoons warm water for soaking

1 (14.5 ounce) can of crushed tomatoes or tomato puree

4 fresh plum tomatoes, deseeded, medium chop

2 tablespoons olive oil for sautéing

2 bay leaves

4 fresh thyme sprigs

4 cups seafood stock

1 organic orange, zested and juiced

2 tablespoons Mirin, or other dry white cooking wine

1 teaspoon salt, plus more to taste

¼ teaspoon freshly ground pepper, or more to taste

Garnish:

¼ cup Italian flat-leaf parsley, chopped

1 tablespoon fresh basil, chopped

Procedure:

1. Keep fish on ice or in the refrigerator. Prep all vegetables.
2. Soak saffron threads in warm water for 10 minutes, set aside.
3. In a large soup pot, sauté onion in olive oil until golden. Stir in garlic and cook 2 minutes.
4. Add leeks, potatoes, carrots, celery, fennel, parsnip, bay leaves, thyme sprigs, and water to cover by three inches. Bring to a boil and cook until potatoes and carrots are soft, about 8 minutes.
5. Add crushed tomatoes or puree, one cup of water, Mirin, saffron threads with soaking liquid, and seafood stock. Cook 15 minutes on medium heat.
6. Add orange zest and juice, and plum tomatoes, stir well.
7. Rinse fish, dry, and rub top with olive oil, salt and pepper. Bake 15 minutes. Halibut may take 5 minutes more.
8. Let fish cool. Cut into 1-inch pieces, almost flaking it. If using shrimp leave whole.
9. Taste the broth and add 1 teaspoon of salt and ¼ teaspoon of pepper, taste and adjust salt, if needed.
10. Gently lay the fish in slowly, stirring once to blend in. Do not over stir, this will break up fish too much. Garnish with the fresh herbs.

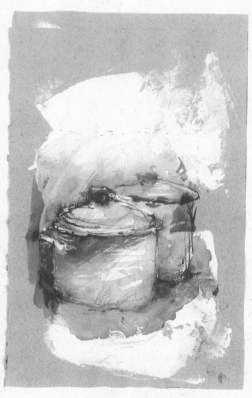

Cook's Notes:

- I suggest using only fresh fish for this dish.
- If using shrimp, purchasing shelled and deveined with tails removed will save time.
- Other fish suggestions: mussels or clams along with two fish choices above, as long as 2 pounds are used.
- Mirin is a Japanese cooking wine. Please see Japanese and Chinese Pantry section in the back of book for a full explanation.
- You may want to add a "bouquet garni" to the soup while cooking. A bouquet garni is a mixture of fresh herbs tied with cooking string or placed in a small linen bag.
- Serve with croutons on top or a side of French bread.
- This soup will stay fresh for 3-4 days.

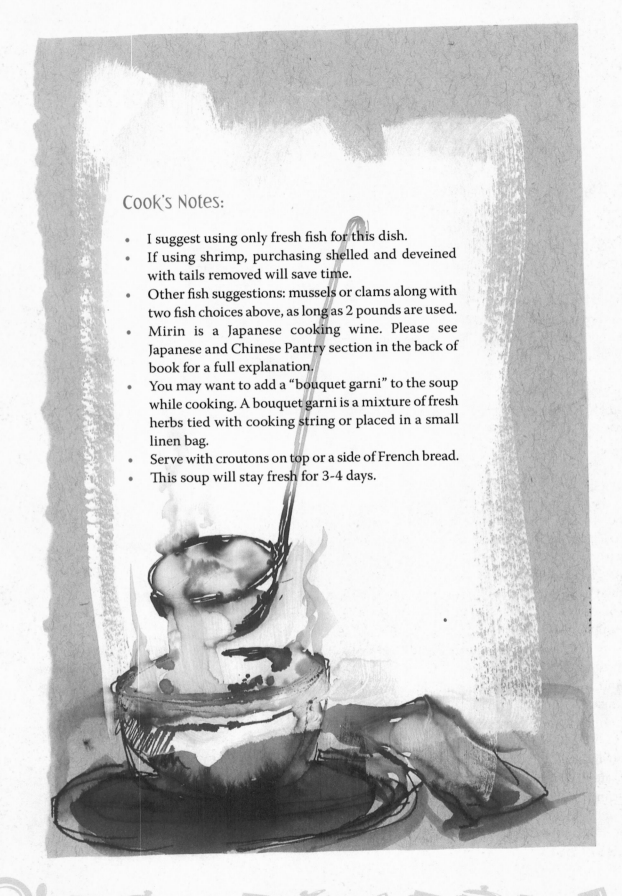

Powerful and Energizing Salads

Empower the warrior in you by creating a variety of nutritious salads weekly.

The following salads all have the elements of crispy, delicious raw vegetables, all bursting with color, texture and an interesting balance of flavors.

All dark leafy greens are abundant in cancer-fighting agents. Greens are high in alkaline minerals too, which promotes excellent PH balance. The big news of kale actually making the cover story in the Sunday magazine section of The New York Times on November 3, 2013 was a thrill for me to see. It's a battle between broccoli sales falling prey to kale sales now, and a big advertising company finding creative ways to bring attention back to broccoli. What the article clearly accomplished for me, was that it brought the attention to all of the green "superfoods". Everyone can use some more greens in their diets. I say to my students, just look outside most of the year, everything is green. It's a green movement going on out there, folks! These super-greens release the feel-good chemicals to the brain. Oxygen is the single most important factor in physical energy, it's also supplied to us through the greens family of hardy vegetables.

The days of kale being the lonely garnish on your plate at restaurants and cafes, to be tossed aside at the end, are for the most part gone. Kale shines now and is very much in the spotlight. Kale is entertainment now too, just turn on YouTube and watch a free video of massaging kale or making fun kale chips with the family.

Our crunchy sweet and tangy cabbage slaw is a power-packed salad with cancer-fighting compounds and hundreds of other naturally occurring phytonutrients. This crunchy salad has a touch of sweetness from caraway seeds and a pungent flavor from horseradish. A real fat-flushing salad. The salad even gets better tasting the next day when all the flavors marry and the cabbage softens.

Our grain salad, Spelt Berry Almond has great character from a whole grain. It's a woody flavor combined with a zesty sweetness from apples, orange zest and juice. Take this salad on a picnic or serve it at a dinner party, it's that versatile. With very little planning you can make whole grains part of your family diet, just as they were 50 years ago, before the modern milling of some of our precious whole grains.

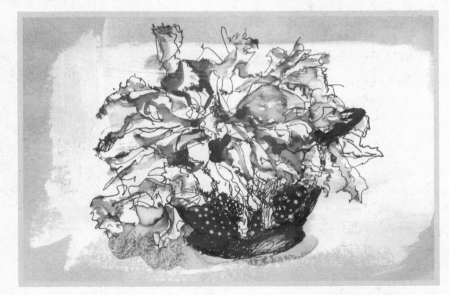

Go green and powerful with these great salads, and engage the energy!

Raw Power Green Salad with Citrus-Fig Salad Dressing

Your daily dose of Mighty Cruciferous Veggies

All greens have different personalities. In this salad, many of them come together for great taste. You'll mix sturdy leaves with interesting textures, sweet and savory vegetable partners and rainbow colors. The end result of all that good stuff is an irresistible crunchy yummy raw salad. (Yes, raw can be yummy). It's unfortunate that most of us don't get enough of the *live enzymes that our bodies need so desperately* – all of which are in this salad. You can restore these enzymes by preparing raw veggies in salads and raw juice drinks. Our diets today have much over-cooked and reheated foods, robbing us of the spark of life that can be found in these foods. The live enzymes within raw foods serve as catalysts to support every human function.

Kale is king here. The ANDI Food Score (Aggregate Nutrient Density Index) rates kale as one of the top 3 foods to eat. Whole Foods Market partnered with The Eat Right America team to establish this score chart (it's a free handout in the store). ANDI scores are calculated by evaluating a range of micronutrients including vitamins, minerals, phytochemicals and antioxidant capacities. Kale has an ANDI score of 1,000, while a carrot is 336, tofu is 37.

Kale is a rich source of bio-available calcium, iron and folic acid and has a full range of antioxidants and bioflavonoids such as Quercetin (which blocks substances involved in allergies, and also protects the stomach lining). I call this health enhancing salad "all -day energy eating." In other words, it smoothes out the highs and lows we can sometimes feel throughout the day by releasing certain chemicals to our brains. Another great bonus with this dark leafy-green veggie is that it is rich in *chlorophyll,* promoting anti-aging properties. It's regenerative and purifying, making it a great chelator of heavy metals and toxins, a natural way to remove them from the body. Eating a steady flow of this green will show up in the form of beautiful skin for you. Not to mention, dark hardy greens can also calm the mind, which makes all our cells smile.

My dearest friend Patti reminds me when she sits down to eat this dish she knows she will be satisfied and have increased energy levels for hours. She feels like she is eating a whole meal not just a green salad. She sometimes will add a ½ cup of the *super grain,* quinoa, on top to make it a rich nutrient packed meal. My Citrus-Fig Salad Dressing has just the right amount of sweetness for this raw salad.

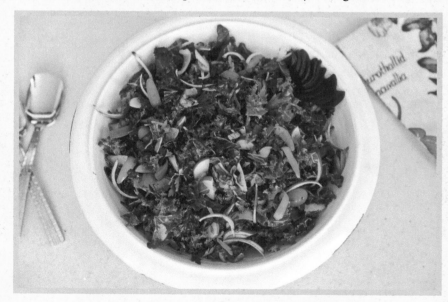

Raw Power Green Salad with Citrus-Fig Salad Dressing

Yield: 6-8 servings

Ingredients:

1 head of curly kale, de-stemmed, leaves torn
1 tablespoon olive oil for massaging kale
1 teaspoon *Celtic Sea Salt*
1 head broccoli florets, small chop, blanched
1 teaspoon sea salt for the above
1 bunch of regular size bok choy, small chop
2 celery stalks, small chop
1 medium cucumber, sliced down center lengthwise, de-seeded, thinly sliced
1 medium carrot, peeled and grated
1 red bell pepper, small chop

½ yellow pepper, thinly sliced
1 small red onion, small chop
2 scallions, white and green parts, thinly sliced
¼ cup Italian flat-leaf parsley, small chop
2 tablespoons cilantro, small chop
¼ cup sugar-free dried cranberries
3 ripe plum tomatoes, deseeded, medium chop
1 ripe avocado, peeled, sliced thin

Optional:
½ cup raw cashews, coarsely chopped

Procedure:

1. Wash and prep all veggies. Keep kale to the side in a separate bowl or strainer. Place the veggies in a medium size bowl and toss gently.
2. Blanch broccoli by dropping into boiling, salted water for 2 minutes. Drain and rinse florets under cold water and place to the side.
3. After washing the kale, shake off excess water. Tear the leaves by hand into bite-size pieces and place in a large mixing bowl. To massage, add 1 tablespoon of olive oil and give the kale a good deep tissue massage for two minutes with some love and a good squeeze. This will give the kale a softer texture and help with digestion. Sprinkle with 1 teaspoon *Celtic Sea Salt*. Massage 30 seconds more.
4. Add the broccoli, bok choy, celery, cucumber, carrots, peppers, onion, scallions, and herbs to the above kale, toss well. Mix in cranberries and add nuts, if using.
5. Slowly blend in half of the Citrus-Fig dressing. If needed, add more being cautious not to make the salad too wet. You want the salad to be firm and crunchy.
6. Add in tomatoes and avocado just before serving.

Cook's Notes:

- Especially in warmer weather, reserve the tomatoes and avocados to add just before serving. This will prevent the salad from becoming mushy.
- *Celtic Sea Salt* is a high-mineral blend, hand-harvested, sun-dried whole salt. I recommend the brand *Selina Naturally*. It comes in *fine* and *course* and is light grey.
- Broccoli can also be raw here, but new-comers to raw salads may fine the above procedure of *blanching* more appealing.
- Always chew raw salads well and slow for better digestion.

Citrus-Fig Salad Dressing

Yield: ¾ cup

Ingredients:

½ cup olive oil plus 2 tablespoons
¼ cup white Champagne vinegar
¼ cup fresh lemon juice
2 teaspoons Dijon mustard
1 tablespoon water

1 tablespoon of *Dalmatia Fig Spread*
1 small shallot, minced
2 tablespoons Italian flat-leaf parsley, small chop
1 teaspoon sea salt
¼ teaspoon ground pepper

Procedure:

1. Whisk first four ingredients well. You can also use a small blender.
2. Slowly blend in the rest of ingredients.
3. Taste and adjust lemon and salt.

Cook's Notes:

- When using this dressing, pour on the bottom of the salad bowl and toss lightly from the bottom just before serving. This will prevent sogginess.
- *Dalmatia Fig Spread* is my favorite. This brand is sold at *Fairway, Whole Foods*, and specialty markets. Choose organic if you can find it.
- Save the dressing in a sealed container in the refrigerator. It will stay fresh up to one week.

A word on Figs:

- Figs made their first appearance in the Holy Scripture "In The Beginning" as clothing for Adam and Eve in the Garden of Eden. The prophet Isaiah used a "lump of figs" to treat the Israelite King Hezekiah, who was sick to death from what was probably a cancer, say biblical scholars. The treatment was successful.
- In Japan, scientists have isolated a cancer-fighting chemical in figs, called Benzaldehyde. It is so potent they've begun adding to cancer medications.
- Besides their sweetness, figs have zero fat and one single fig has 40 calories. According to one USDA study, figs have the power to decrease appetite and improve weight loss efforts. They are high in calcium, magnesium and potassium.
- Fig cooking water is excellent for sore throats.
- In baking, figs are darling as a roll-up cookie or bar cookie or tart with other fruit. How about Paul Newman's famous cookies - Fig Newton's anyone?

Crunchy Sweet and Tangy Slaw

Get ready to clean up the pipes and feel great. It's amazing that a salad that is so, so healthy can be so scrumptious. I love to serve this rainbow of color salad in small bowls before a meal that has a good portion of beef, lamb or chicken in it. Cabbage can help neutralize that fat.

You'll be surprised to experience so many different tastes and countless applications for one of the world's oldest recorded foods, cabbage. This vegetable is part of an exceptional family, the *cruciferous family*, that are touted for their powerful healing compounds that exhibit cancer fighting properties, partially against lung, colon, stomach and breast cancers. This nutritional powerhouse is high in fiber, which makes it a great fat flusher.

Allergy sufferers can really benefit from eating cabbage. The nutrient and special compounds in cabbage clean up mucus build-ups, colds, and sinus problems. A great source of chromium, cabbage can also regulate insulin and blood sugar levels. This means it's an anti-fat nutrient. Cooking can destroy some of the antioxidants, so do eat it raw.

Cabbage juice has been known to kill cancer cells, with its cancer fighting nutrients, vitamin c, and two phytochemicals, sulforaphane and indoles. These two compounds help to detoxify the body, ridding it of excess estrogen. This is great news for women suffering from PMS. A number of studies show that women who include cabbage regularly in their diet can reduce their risk of breast cancer by 45 percent by just adding at least three-½ cup servings per week.

Cabbage can add a wholesome flair to your tossed salad. Why not tuck some in a burrito?

This nutritional superstar will also give you beautiful skin. It is a secret from Asian women for centuries. The horseradish in the recipe also helps with sinus issues and allergies. This bitter herb used at the Passover Seder is an excellent detoxifier capable of killing germs.

So get your cabbage on and be a clean machine!!

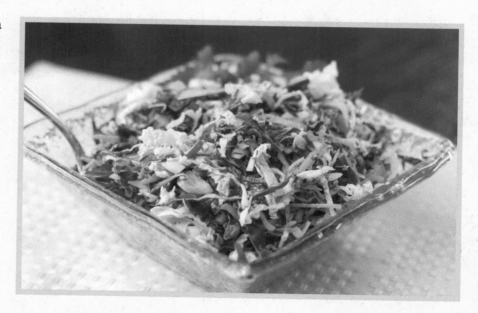

Crunchy Sweet and Tangy Slaw

Yield: 8 servings

Ingredients:

¾ head green cabbage, thinly sliced
⅓ head purple cabbage, thinly sliced
1 large carrot, grated
1 red pepper, thinly sliced
½ yellow pepper, thinly sliced
1 small red onion, small chop

3 scallions, white and green parts, thinly sliced
2 tablespoons Italian flat-leaf parsley, finely chopped
2 teaspoons caraway seeds
1 tablespoon fresh dill, finely chopped, or 1 ½
    teaspoon dried
Sea salt and freshly ground pepper to taste

Dressing:

2 tablespoons sesame oil
3 tablespoons apple cider vinegar
2 tablespoons honey
¼ cup dairy-free mayonnaise, such as *Vegenaise*

1 teaspoon Dijon mustard
1 tablespoon prepared horseradish sauce
1 teaspoon sea salt
¼ teaspoon freshly ground pepper

Procedure:

1. In a large mixing bowl add the sliced cabbages, carrots, peppers, onion, scallions, parsley, caraway seeds, dill, salt and pepper. Mix to incorporate all.
2. In a separate small bowl, whisk the oil and vinegar to blend together. Add the rest of dressing ingredients and stir to combine.
3. Toss the dressing with the veggies and let mixture sit for 10 minutes. Taste and adjust flavors. If you feel it needs more of a "tangy" taste, whisk together 2 teaspoons vinegar with 1 teaspoon horseradish sauce and add to the slaw. Adjust salt.

Cook's Notes:

- Fresh horseradish is always best to use when in season (Fall and Winter months).
- If using fresh horseradish, peel and grate a small piece using the larger holes of your grater. Start with two teaspoons, then, when adjusting tastes in step #3, if you prefer a more pungent taste, use 1 teaspoon more.
- I prefer *Gold's* horseradish, which can be found in most supermarkets.
- If you prefer a creamier slaw, add an extra 2 tablespoons of the non-dairy mayo.
- This slaw will last up to 5 days. It tastes amazing mixed with your favorite salad.

Bountiful Spelt Berry Almond Salad with Citrus Vinaigrette

Spelt Berries are major league players in the health field stadium and the payoffs are powerfully delicious.

An exceptional heirloom whole grain that keeps its glory through the test of time, spelt berries originated in the Near East 8,000 years ago. The jewel like berries are the dried seeds of the plant unaltered. A super grain with a substantial variety of vitamins and minerals, it is considered serious nutrition yet, in this recipe, it's simply delightful with waves of sweetness from almonds, oranges and golden raisins.

This salad is an interesting alchemy providing both energizing and calming effects on the senses, after eating and digestion. This "staff of life grain" has a hundred years of research behind it which show that whole grains have slow-release complex carbohydrates. This allows the body to need less insulin than refined carbs need for digestion. This is great news for diabetics. This slow release of sugars also helps regulate the rate of the release for specific hormones and other important nutrients. The experts are recommending the use of whole grains and other high fiber foods such as lentils, split peas, and beans for prevention of heart, liver, colon and kidney disease.

All of the above leads me to this short story: I demonstrated this recipe in a cooking workshop with my assistant Karen and a group of young savvy moms. These moms were looking to educate and empower themselves and their families via the knowledge of cooking healthier, life supporting foods.

There were some samples left after the workshop and Karen served a small portion of this salad to her friend Katrina who had stopped by. Katrina had a cupful for breakfast with Karen and ran all day doing her many errands, then driving her kids to sports after school and basically multi-tasking. At the end of this day she still had more energy to go. The next day she called Karen and asked, "What was that salad and where can I find the recipe?" Now I make sure to include this recipe in all my workshops. This brilliant surge of energy comes from eating *whole foods*.

Contributing to the goodness of this salad are almonds, which are a great source of protein. These jewels are one of the only nuts to alkalize the body and at the same time supply us with important fats, called Essential Fatty Acids. Their special talents are to produce life energy in our body from food substances and move that energy through our systems.

The apples are a great source of protein (yes, apples have protein.) When you cut an organic apple open, it will start to brown shortly. This is the evidence of a live food source. Buyer beware, apples are high on the dirty dozen list so choose organic to be free of preservatives and pesticides.

Go with the grain and fuel your body with this abundant salad and earn points for stamina and endurance. Get a make-ahead game plan and cook the spelt berries a day before.

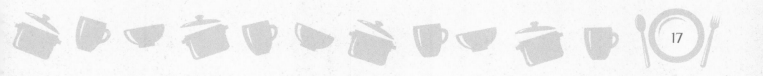

Spelt Berry Almond Salad with Citrus Vinaigrette

Yield: 6 servings

Ingredients:

1 cup uncooked spelt berries
1 small red onion, small chop
1 medium carrot, peeled and grated
2 stalks celery, small chop
1 granny smith apple, peeled, small chop
½ red pepper, small chop
½ cup golden raisins
½ cup almonds, small chop
¼ cup Italian flat-leaf parsley, small chop
1 organic orange, zested and juiced
1 teaspoon sea salt
¼ teaspoon ground pepper

Dressing:

3 tablespoons olive oil
2 tablespoons apple cider vinegar
Juice from the orange
1 teaspoon sea salt

Garnish:

2 scallion's white and green parts, medium chop

Procedure:

1. For the spelt berries: Rinse and drain. Soak overnight or 2 -3 hours in hot water. In a 6-quart saucepan, bring 7 cups of water to a boil. Add drained berries and cook on medium for 30 minutes if soaked overnight, and 45 minutes if soaked 2-3 hours. Berries should be soft and crunchy when done. Drain and set aside to cool.
2. In a large mixing bowl combine the onion, carrot, celery, apple, red pepper, raisins, almonds, parsley, orange zest, salt, and pepper. Toss well.
3. Whisk the dressing ingredients together. Add to the above salad with the spelt berries.
4. Chill salad for 30 minutes in the refrigerator before serving for flavors to blend.

Cook's Notes:

- Soaking the hard berries is ideal because it helps with the digestion process, however you will still have a delicious salad if you can't soak. If golden raisins are not available, regular raisins will do.
- To zest an orange you can use a small grater, zester or micro-plane. I like to zest over wax paper or the actual bowl.
- Use only organic citrus to zest. Our Government allows the use of many pesticides on citrus fruits because they don't think people ever use the skin.

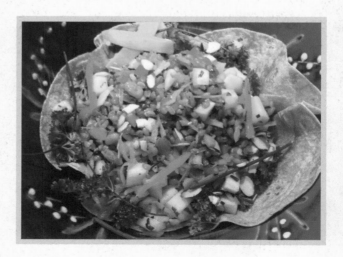

The Possibilities with Protein

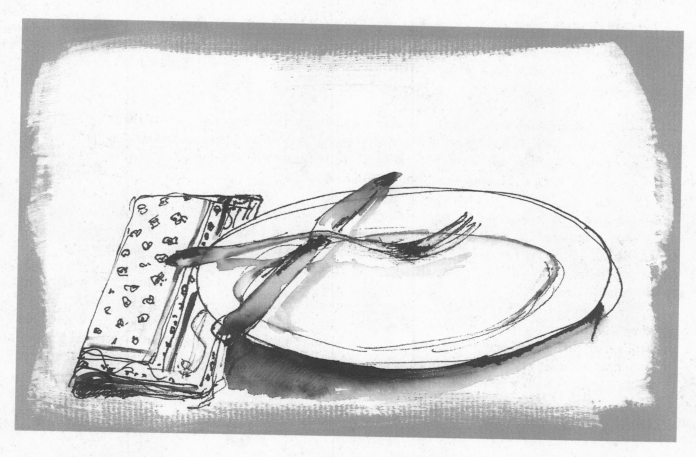

As a vegetarian cook I can still appreciate quality animal and fish protein in my diet. In a meal with an animal protein, I always combine a variety of colorful nutritious vegetables, spices, garnished with fresh herbs such as parsley, or cilantro, dill or basil. A fresh, crisp salad is always on the side. Experts in nutrition suggest rotating your proteins daily. For me, it always works well.

Certain holidays in my Italian culture are associated with different animal proteins and cuts of meat. In Italy, lamb symbolizes the first days of spring and is served at the Easter celebration. Every culture in this world has their unique story, similar to this one.

We recently celebrated Christmas at my daughter's and her husband beautifully prepared a prime rib of beef. The dish was surrounded by a few healthy green crisp vegetables and a fresh salad. These side dishes definitely helped in the digestion of the meat and chewing the meat well is also critical to digestion.

In Asian cultures, raw ginger in many forms such as salad dressing, picked ginger, and ginger juice is eaten before the protein meal to neutralize the fat. This sounds so logical and purifying to me, restoring balance and aiding in the digestion.

The Rainbow Turkey Veggie Loaf is a practical staple meal in my house. The fat in the meat is balanced by the rainbow of colored vegetables. The Chicken Meatballs are tasty and tender and have instant popularity with kids and adults. A good amount of fresh parsley adds a healthy ingredient to this chicken dish.

I really feel grateful when I purchase my Wild Salmon at my neighborhood's fish store. Whether I just broil or grill it, it always makes me feel satisfied and strong. My experience with many families with young children who don't want to eat fish is to cook the salmon in a burger or croquette form. It happens to be a favorite for adults too. It is a great way to get everyone to experience this fish.

My Sardine Salad recipe surprises everyone. I suggest you start with the ones packed with their skin and bones in olive oil. However, if you doubt whether you will like them, I do give you permission to start with the skinless and boneless sardines. They can be a stepping stone for you to graduate to the bone building ones, that is, with the skin and bones intact. If you eat tuna fish you will enjoy them.

Remember that protein is a vital nutrient essential to our health. All the tissues of the body are built and repaired with protein. The antibodies of the immune system, most hormones, and the hemoglobin of red blood cells have protein as their base component. Proteins help to repair and replace new tissue, transport oxygen and nutrients in our blood and cells, they help to make antibodies and regulate the necessary balance of water and acids.

The theme in America is "more is better." Contrary to belief, too much of even a good thing may not always be good for you. Therefore, eat your animal protein in moderation and always have good fiber sources in your diet. When shopping, make an effort to buy organic beef, chicken, turkey and lamb. In this essential food category please shop smarter to find better meats.

Rainbow Turkey Veggie Loaf

This recipe was created in 1984 when my two children were living and working in New York City. I wanted it to be a comfort food that would yield a few meals for them. It works for a busy lifestyle and it worked for them. It has become a favorite of so many families since.

When we had *The Health Conscious Café*, the Turkey Veggie Loaf was sold from our establishment on a weekly basis to a deli, two health food stores and a gym (that served food in their café). It warms my heart to think that one recipe traveled so far and nourished so many people.

I enjoyed how the businessmen would come in at lunch and would say, "give me that turkey loaf with the works." It has so much less saturated fat than the classic meatloaf. It's totally worth the time it takes to make, although you can certainly prep it out the day before. It slices beautifully and makes a dynamic sandwich on rye bread with Russian dressing, green goddess dressing or just avocado and lettuce and a juicy tomato. It's so pleasing to the eye with the rainbow colors from the many veggies. It truly deserves its title as a *comfort food*.

Mom's you can get your young children to enjoy this loaf. Make it in mini loaf pans, they will love having their own loaf, even they will be impressed.

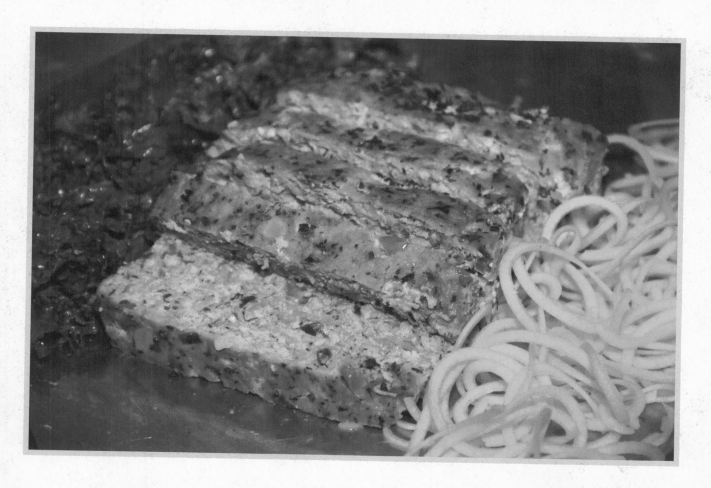

Rainbow Turkey Veggie Loaf

Yield: 2 standard loaf pans or one large

Ingredients:

1 small Spanish onion, small chop

6 garlic cloves, minced

2 tablespoons olive oil

1 teaspoon ground oregano

1 teaspoon ground thyme

1 teaspoon ground basil

1 teaspoon sea salt

¼ teaspoon freshly ground black pepper

1 tablespoon Tamari (wheat-free soy sauce)

1 medium carrot, peeled and grated

¾ cup crushed or chopped tomatoes (using canned is fine)

½ red, yellow and orange pepper, small chop

2 organic large eggs or 1 egg and 2 egg whites

1½ pounds hormone-free ground white turkey breast meat

½ pound hormone-free ground dark turkey meat

¼ cup Italian Parmesan cheese, grated

½ cup Italian flat-leaf parsley, small chop

1 cup Italian-style breadcrumbs (no MSG or preservatives)

1 teaspoon salt

½ teaspoon ground pepper

Procedure:

1. Preheat oven to 350 degrees, lightly oil loaf pan(s).
2. In a medium-size frying pan or saucepan, sauté the onion in olive oil until golden. Add the garlic and stir 1-2 minutes until fragrant. Add spices and stir one minute.
3. Add the Tamari, tomatoes, carrots and peppers and cook 1 minute. Be cautious to not allow peppers to get soft.
4. In a large mixing bowl place the turkey meat, eggs, and the sauté mixture. Stir well to blend. Add the breadcrumbs, cheese, and parsley. Mix until just blended.
5. Bake for 30 minutes uncovered, then cover with foil loosely and cook 15 minutes more. It must be firm to the touch on top. If not, cook 10 more minutes covered. Cool completely before slicing.

Cook's Notes:

- Look for gluten-free breadcrumbs, if necessary.
- You can omit cheese, if needed. The loaf will still be delicious.
- My suggestion is for busy Mom's to prep all veggies the day before… it's good time management!
- The loaf will stay fresh up to 4-5 days but I promise it will not last that long.
- Roasted sweet potatoes or brown rice make a great side. Bone building veggies such as mustard greens or collards make this the total package.

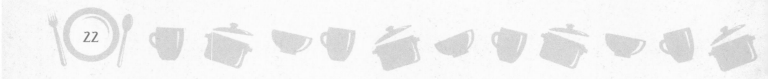

Be Sardine Savvy

Want to know my very best kept secret for achieving optimal energy, productive work and operates as a big anti-aging bonus?

It's a little tin filled with full flavored, rich and meaty fishes called sardines. They're one of world's healthiest convenience foods, and easy on the pocketbook. I love them for the way they make me feel, and trust me, they can appeal to almost everyone when complimented with delicious condiments. We love them tossed with toasted pine nuts, parsley, tomato sauce, onions and cooked brown rice stuffed into a par-boiled red pepper.

If my hubby brings home pizza, I take a piece and smash some of my sardines, with a back of a spoon, right into the cheese, with some fresh basil or parsley. What a feast for me! Some people eat them right out of the can, while aficionados age them in private cellars and crack open vintage tins to celebrate special occasions.

Sardines used to school in great numbers off the Italian island of Sardinia. Hence the name. Sardines have been a staple protein in many cultures on many continents. Sardines have been shipped out to troops around the world for two centuries. Their rich protein delivers stamina.

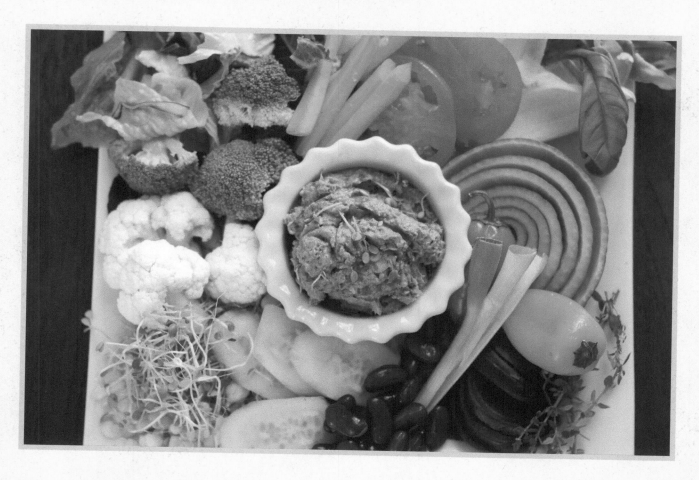

Sardines are "Heart- Healthy."

* They are chocked full of heart healthy Omega-3 fatty acids. They are rich in Purine protein.
* They promote a healthy immune system by providing Co-Q10, a potent antioxidant that protects your cells from damaging free radicals; restores youthful vitality, high in Vitamin D, and are bone builders.
* They are high in Nucleic Acids (they deteriorate as we age) and enhance the quality of our DNA and RNA
* Sardines are richest in Nitric Oxide, a vasodilator that helps control blood flow to every part of your body.
* It has also been shown that sardines enhance cellular metabolism and energy production.

On a recent trip to Ellis Island – the entry point for my own relatives and my husband's - we were so excited to do the tour, learn about all the details and then end up at the end in a quaint replica of the Café area. The original menu was in three languages. I was jumping for joy to see sardines on the menu for just $.02 cents

It makes me feel good to know that our grandparents, arriving hungry, tired, a bit stressed with not too much money, could choose sardines for the healthiest lunch or dinner and certainly be nourished.

Celebrate life - eat sardines. They will nourish and help support your healthy lifestyle!

My Very Savvy Sardine Plate (My Longevity Plate)

Yield: 4 servings

Ingredients:

2 cans of sardines in olive oil, with skin and bones
(see resource list below)

¼ cup walnuts, roasted, small chop

2 ripe avocados, mashed

½ of a small red onion, small chop

2 celery stalks, small chop

¼ cup Italian flat-leaf parsley, small chop

3 teaspoons chopped sweet relish

2 teaspoons fresh lemon juice (one lemon)

2 tablespoons dairy-free mayonnaise, such as
Vegenaise

1 teaspoon sea salt

3 plum tomatoes, deseeded, small chop

Plating suggestions:

1. Pungent greens like watercress and arugula, sweet lettuces like bib or red leaf, sweet raw veggies like carrots, and chopped jicama.
2. Italian olives, roasted corn, and cannellini or black beans.
3. Steamed beets and a sprinkle of dried unsweetened cranberries are divine.

Serving Suggestion:

- Serve with flatbreads or a multi grain baguette, alongside of a chunk of imported Parmesan cheese.

Procedure:

1. Preheat oven to 350 degrees.
2. Drain the oil from the sardine cans. Mash them into a medium sized mixing bowl.
3. Roast walnuts for 6-8 minutes. Cool and chop.
4. In a medium bowl mix together the mashed avocado, onion, celery, parsley, relish and walnuts.
5. In a separate bowl, whisk together the lemon juice and the mayonnaise. Stir in the sea salt. Add mixture to the sardines and vegetables and fold in the plum tomatoes.
6. Taste and adjust lemon juice and mayonnaise by adding a teaspoon of each, if needed.
7. Garnish plates with above suggestions.

Cook's Notes:

- These are my favorite choices for authentic sardines: *Bela Sardines*; *Wild Vital Choice Sardines*; *Wild Planet, Wild Sardines*; *Crown Prince, Wild Caught Sardines*. Some Companies will package other soft-boned fish and different species of fish to be called sardines. There's a very different taste profile between a true sardine and the other species of "sardines." Portugal produces delicious sardines from clean waters, so look to buy sardines from Portugal.
- Some of the above sardines can be packed in mustard sauce, tomato sauce, hot sauce, or even smoked naturally.
- My husband occasionally will have a sardine sandwich for breakfast, on sliced fresh pumpernickel bread with a juicy tomato, lettuce, slices of red onion and a splash of the vegan mayonnaise. We think it's a rich way to start the day.

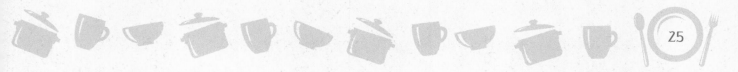

My Magical Meatball Story

In my family, meatballs of any sort, "Rule." Italian flavored meatballs are part of our Cultural Heritage. The Italian mix of the meat was always, veal, pork, and beef. Now my family will be just as satisfied with less saturated fat and I can substitute that mixture with chicken or turkey meat.

Rolling and cooking the meatballs: One day before Mother's Day many years ago I was preparing to have my immediate family over. I had not seen either of my children for about two months or so, and in anticipation of them coming, I was starting to fill up with much joy (that is, I could feel my heart center pumping up with that joy and gratitude) . I was blessed to be able to purchase the finest organic wholesome foods around town and have the day off to cook without pressure for time. I kicked off my shoes and put on great music, and my beautiful intention was to make the best meatballs ever for my loved ones.

The sunshine was glowing in through my kitchen window and I started thinking of the family, "**The Familia**". As I was rolling the meatballs, which by the way starting smelling divine, something magical happened to me. I literally felt I was lifted out of my body, and just my soul was exposed. Runners have explained this feeling as runners' high, where all those great endorphins are released.

According to Deepak Chopra, a well-known medical doctor and great spiritual leader, the unbelievable, phenomenal feeling I was experiencing while cooking relates to parts of the Hindu Veda. This is sacred Hindu scripture and the texts that deal with self-realization and one's understanding of the ultimate nature of reality. The passage below was adapted by Deepak Chopra: "The Spontaneous Fulfillment of Desire. (Three Rivers Press)"

> According to Vedanta, (one of the world's most ancient philosophies and is the philosophical foundation of Hinduism) there are seven states of consciousness. Each of the seven states of consciousness represents an increase in our experience of synchronicity, and each progressive state move us closer to the ideal of enlightenment.
>
> Most of us only experience the first three, sleeping, dreaming, and wakefulness. The fourth state of consciousness occurs when we actually glimpse the soul when we become aware of the observer inside us. This state of consciousness occurs during meditation.
>
> The fifth state of consciousness is called cosmic consciousness. In this state, your spirit can observe your material body. Your awareness goes beyond simply being awake in your body, and beyond simply glimpsing the soul, to being awake and alert to your place as part of the infinite spirit.
>
> The observer can observe the body while it's dreaming and simultaneously observe the dream. The same experience occurs in waking consciousness. You have two qualities to your awareness, local and nonlocal, at the same time. Your intuition increases. Your creativity and insight increases.

The sixth state of consciousness is called divine consciousness. In this state, the witness becomes more and more awake. You not only feel the presence of spirit in yourself, but you start to feel that same spirit in all other beings.

The seventh state, the ultimate goal, is called unity consciousness, or enlightenment. The spirit in the perceiver and the spirit in that which is perceived merge and become one. When this happens, you see the whole world as an extension of your own being.

In this state *miracles are commonplace*, but they are not even necessary because the infinite realm of possibility is available in every moment. *You transcend life. You transcend death. You are the spirit that always was and always will be.*

Wow, how profound is that? I believe each of us can embody this beautiful, amazing passage in our own lives, in our own kitchens preparing the family meal, not just for a holiday but for any day or night of the week. You use your hands to cut and chop and clean but with endless possibilities of the magical moments that can happen at every thought of your loved ones. You can transcend the commonplace and reach a place to connect to cosmic consciousness or enlightenment as I did, in the fifth state, of consciousness. Believe!

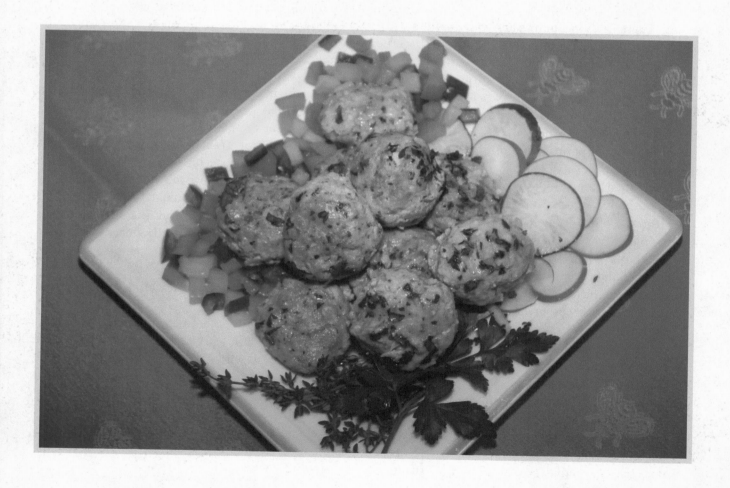

Melt In Your Mouth Mini Chicken Meatballs

Yield: 40 mini or 20 regular size meatballs

Ingredients:

2 medium shallots, minced
6 garlic cloves, minced
2 tablespoons olive oil for sautéing
1 teaspoon ground oregano
1 teaspoon ground thyme
½ teaspoon ground fennel
1 pound free-range ground chicken breast meat
1 teaspoon sea salt
¼ ground fresh pepper
½ cup plain breadcrumbs (no MSG)

½ cup Italian flat-leaf parsley, small chop
2 large eggs, slightly beaten
1 tablespoon whole milk
1 tablespoon ketchup
¾ cup grated Romano cheese
1 ½ cups free-ranged low-sodium chicken broth
¼ cup grape seed or safflower oil (for high heat)
2 tablespoons freshly grated Parmesan cheese, to top
3 tablespoons fresh basil, medium chop

Procedure:

1. In a small frying pan, sauté the shallots until golden. Add garlic and stir 2 minutes to become fragrant. Add spices to incorporate.
2. In a large bowl mix together the ground chicken with the breadcrumbs, parsley, eggs, milk, ketchup, Romano cheese, salt and pepper. Blend well but don't over mix. Mixture will be sticky.
3. Using a tablespoon, scoop out balls onto a sheet pan lined with wax paper.
4. With oiled hands roll the balls between to form a smooth, mini meatball. Transfer balls to a plate.
5. Heat the oil in a large sauté pan over medium to high heat. Working in two batches, add the meatballs when the oil starts to sizzle. Have another plate ready for the first batch.
6. Brown the meat on one side and roll with spoon carefully to the other to side, about 3 minutes each side. Total cooking time is 6-8 minutes depending on if your stove top is gas or electric heat. Meatballs tend to stick so work fast.
7. Pour out cooking oil, and wipe out pan with a paper towel. Keep the heat on medium to high. Add the broth and bring to a boil. Add meatballs carefully then lower to a simmer.
8. Cook meatballs for 20 minutes only, turn off heat. If serving immediately, plate the meatballs in an appropriate platter with a lip for juice. Garnish while hot with the Parmesan cheese. Add fresh cut basil to the dish to finish it.

Cook's Notes:

- You can make your own breadcrumbs for this recipe. *To make breadcrumbs,* preheat oven to 250 degrees. For 1 cup breadcrumbs, place 12 (¼-inch-thick) slices of French bread or a multi-grain baguette in one layer on a baking sheet and bake 15 minutes, or until crisp and lightly browned (dry bread will be done more quickly). Let cool to room temperature. Pulse the bread in a food processor fitted with the metal blade until reduced to relatively uniform crumbs. (Store at room temperature, in an airtight container for up to 2 weeks.)
- If you're gluten-free, you can use gluten-free breadcrumbs here.
- Here are two ideas for great meals for the family: Sauté some dark leafy green veggies, like kale or collard greens with a small piece of red onion. Cut the meatballs in half, almost to look like a small bite and toss the meatballs gently into the sauté. Top off with favorite dressing.
- You can tuck them in a pita pocket halved or a burrito, add lettuce and sprouts and a tomato for a yummy wrap.

This recipe was adapted from *Giada De Laurentiis' Chicken Meatball Recipe.*

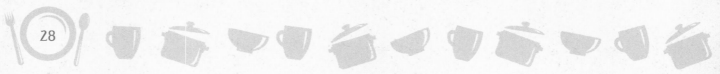

Wild Wonderful Salmon Burgers

For over twenty years my private clients and customers, friends and family members love these wild ones.

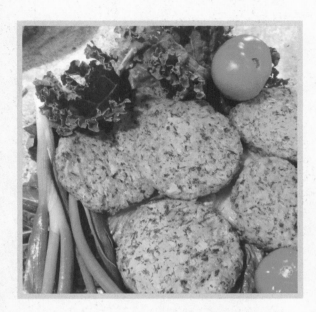

They are an interesting symphony of healthy ingredients paired with a mild salmon flavor (meaning they are not fishy tasting). They are versatile and satisfying to use as appetizers at your next casual gathering or special holiday. My most picky friends and clients have told me that they are not even sure they are eating fish. The leeks and shallots caramelize to sweetness. The sweet potato and fresh dill & parsley crown the dish.

Use your mini chopper or Cuisinart to breeze through the prep. When baked together they are soft yet hearty, and that makes them a great comfort food. They are very economical too. This recipe yields 11 burgers or 22 croquettes and only 1 ¼ pounds of the fish. They freeze well also, but I promise they are usually eaten first and that's a good thing for everyone's healthier heart and long life.

Wild salmon has the highest amounts of EPA/DHA. These are essential fatty acids that our bodies do not create; we need to supplement our diets in order to get them. This meaty tasting fish is also high in Omega-3's, as well as nucleic acids, which are necessary for good cellular health, promoting healthy arteries. One fascinating new area of health benefits involves the high protein and amino acid content in salmon that supports joint cartilage, insulin effectiveness and controls chronic inflammation in the gut. Let's not forget an added bonus for "anti-aging" factors.

Buyer beware, not all salmon is created equal. I suggest purchasing this fish at your neighborhood seafood store. It makes sense to ask lots of questions because chances are you will see at least three different types of salmon, however there are six types consumed in the US. The three different types of wild-caught Pacific salmon that are considered the best are: King (Chinook); Sockeye (Red); and Silver (Coho). The last three types are; Pink and Chum, and these two are usually canned and often sold to foreign markets, the sixth type, Atlantic, is primarily farmed raised. Farmed salmon, which should be clearly labeled these days, has high concentrations of antibiotics, pesticides, and lower levels of healthy nutrients. There are many wonderful organizations that are steering customers and businesses toward sustainably fished seafood. Two such organizations are; "Monterey Bay Aquarium *Seafood Watch*" and "Blue Ocean Institute."

Wild Salmon Burgers or Croquettes

Yield: 11 large burgers or 22 croquettes

Ingredients:

1¼ pounds of wild salmon

2 large or 3 medium sweet potatoes or yams, cooked and mashed

2 teaspoons organic butter

2 tablespoons olive oil for sauté

½ cup shallots, (about 3 medium), minced

3 medium leeks, white parts only, small chop

1 cup chopped celery

1 yellow pepper, small chop

¼ cup seasoned breadcrumbs (no MSG)

½ cup Italian flat-leaf parsley, small chop

¼ cup fresh dill, small chop

1½ teaspoon sea salt

¼ teaspoon freshly ground pepper

3 large egg whites, slightly beaten

1 tablespoon dairy-free mayonnaise, such as *Vegenaise*

1 teaspoon Dijon mustard

Garnish:

Wedges of lemon

Procedure:

1. Preheat oven to Broil Hi - 500 degrees.
2. Place salmon under the broiler for 8 minutes. The top will start to get crispy. Lower the temperature to 350 degrees and cook for another 9 minutes. Set aside to cool.
3. In a 400 degree oven, cook sweet potatoes with skins on for 40-45 minutes, until soft. Cool. Take skins off and mash with the butter. You can also steam with skins on in a steamer basket until soft, about 15-20 minutes. Take off skins and mash. Set aside.
4. In a medium-size frying pan or saucepan, sauté shallots in olive oil stirring constantly until slightly crispy. Raise heat to high. Add leeks, cook 1 minute. Add celery and yellow pepper and stir constantly, about 1 minute. You want the sauté to be a bit crispy, not burned.
5. Set oven to 375 degrees. Prepare a sheet pan with natural parchment paper.
6. In a medium sized mixing bowl shred salmon with a fork into fine pieces. Watch for any tiny white bones. Add the mashed potatoes, the sauté mixture, breadcrumbs, parsley, dill, salt and pepper, stir well to incorporate.
7. In a small bowl whisk the eggs with the mayonnaise and Dijon. Add to the salmon bowl and blend well. The whole mixture will look wet. If too wet (where it doesn't form a burger when you shape it) add 2 tablespoons of bread crumbs.
8. With an ice cream scooper, a burger form, or with your hands, shape into patties and place on oiled baking sheet with space between each patty to turn over. Bake for 15 minutes, flip them, and cook 12 more minutes. Burgers should be slightly crispy. Follow the same procedure for croquettes, using a melon baller or a full tablespoon. Cooking time is 10 minutes on each side. Allow to cool on a wire rack for 20 minutes.
9. Store in a glass container or wax paper bags.

Cook's Notes:

- You'll need to use a flat ceramic or glass baking dish to use under the broiler.
- Store salmon burgers in glass containers or brown wax paper bags. They freeze well.
- Wild salmon is best. You can use other types as long as the fish is not farm-raised.
- Leeks are sandy. Be sure to soak in a bowl and then rinse through a strainer.
- Use a small chopper to mince the shallots.

Developing Your Asian Kitchen with Delight

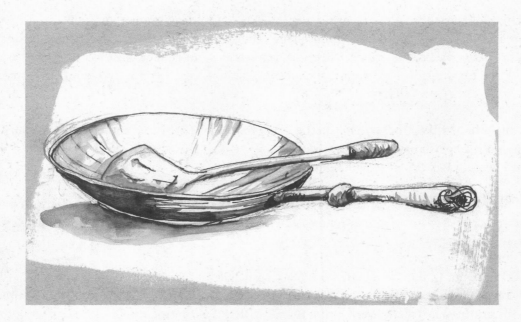

The following are three of my favorite Asian recipes. They truly demonstrate much creativity and mindfulness in this style of cooking. If you've never tried this kind of cooking, it's fun to learn, and with practice you'll build your skills.

Chinese and Japanese food has a multi-layered depth of flavor and texture. To get to the finished product, simply requires organizing the essential ingredients.

First you always need to read through the recipes and be sure that you understand the timing of any unfamiliar techniques. The ingredients can be found on my Japanese and Chinese Pantry lists in the back of the book. What a great adventure to learn the preparation and techniques of the Stir-fry and for making hand-crafted Chinese rolls.

In this special style of cooking, the bulk of the time is spent in preparation and not in the actual cooking time, which usually goes by quickly. Have fun starting to collect the appropriate little vessels (prep bowls) to organize the ingredients to be cooked. These bowls, in all shapes and colors and textures, are now sold everywhere.

Keep in mind that some of the fresh ingredients, such as Bok Choy, Watercress and Cabbage, are part of a powerful food group called *Cruciferous* vegetables, which boost longevity. The magical root, ginger, and lots of potent garlic, herbs and spices, noodles from mung beans and whole edamame, grace these dishes.

Nutritionally speaking, these Asian dishes are packed with nutrient-rich power. Our bodies need to rotate different foods to spark the life in the body. So get ready to recreate these essential Asian dishes with confidence. Enjoy the sizzle of the ingredients, and get inspired to know and feel the *Yin* and *Yang* of my favorite Asian dishes.

You can do this! It's my hope for you to expand your repertoire of easy techniques for East-Meets-West meals.

Baked Chinese Spring Rolls for a Symphony of Tastes

Chinese Spring Rolls are one of my favorite creations. The old adage states that good things come in small packages and, in this case, it could not be more true. They're a bundle of sweet flavors and crunchy textures in a crisp skin that is baked, *not fried*. A drop of pure sesame oil rubbed on the roll before baking creates crispness, not like the ones in the Chinese restaurants that are fried in undesirable oil. This version satisfies the palette, just ask my many clients.

Chinese Spring Rolls are like a little stir-fry in the wrapper. My favorite is the combo of ginger, garlic, scallions, and coriander with a splash of sweet Mirin (rice cooking wine), paired with stir-fry vegetables. You also can be resourceful here and use up any vegetables that will perish soon in your refrigerator.

Spring rolls, like veggie burgers, are friendly foods that offer fundamental nutrition. You can pack them up for a light lunch or serve as an appetizer for a casual friend's dinner. Some interesting dips and sauces make a perfect compliment to the rolls.

I have served these, cut in half on the diagonal, with a beautiful garnish at many a dinner party or for very special occasions. One that comes to mind so dearly is my daughter Melina's 30th birthday in Manhattan in her friend Steve's beautiful apartment overlooking the East River. The spring rolls were plated on a sterling silver pedestal platter and garnished with edible layers of colorful vegetables and sprouts. What a beautiful and fun presentation that made for her special evening.

Everyone can enjoy the soulful experience of making these Chinese Spring Rolls anytime of the year, for any occasion. Hopefully, they will inspire you to create a beautiful garnish and an attractive table setting to instill a sense of harmony and beauty at the table.

Baked Chinese Spring Rolls with Sesame-Ginger Dipping Sauce

Yield: 24 appetizer or 12 entrée rolls

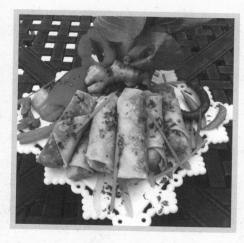

Ingredients:

1 package of egg roll wrappers or spring roll skins

¾ cup mung bean pasta (also called cellophane noodles)

4 tablespoons sesame oil, 1 tablespoon reserved

1 small Spanish onion, thinly sliced into half-moons

4 large garlic cloves, minced

2-inch knob of fresh ginger, minced to measure 2 tablespoons

6 scallions, white and green parts, thinly sliced, divided

1 teaspoon ground coriander

2 tablespoons Mirin

2 cups thinly sliced Nappa cabbage

1½ cups thinly sliced Swiss chard

1 cup thinly sliced fresh spinach

1 large carrot, peeled and grated

¼ cup Tamari (wheat-free soy sauce) mixed with ¼ cup water

¼ cup chopped cilantro

1½ cups of sprouts, such as sunflower or pea

Procedure:

1. Allow egg roll wrappers to come to room temperature.

2. Prepare a baking sheet with natural parchment paper.

3. In a 3 to 4-quart pot bring 4 cups of water to a boil. Drop mung bean noodles in boiling water and cook for 2 minutes. Drain and chop into small pieces.

4. In a large frying pan, skillet, or wok, sauté onion in sesame oil until golden. Add garlic, stir 1 minute. Add ginger and half the scallions, stirring for 1 minute. Sprinkle in coriander, and mix together.

5. Increase the heat to high and add the Mirin to sizzle. Add cabbage, chard, spinach, and carrots. Stir well.

6. Stir in the Tamari-water mixture and cover. Keep the heat on high for 3 minutes to steam the veggies without wilting.

7. Remove cover, stir and lower heat. Add cilantro and noodles and the remaining scallions.

8. In a medium-size tight-mesh strainer, and over a medium bowl, drain the vegetable mixture, pressing mixture down with back of wooden spoon, to release a sauce or "gravy." Reserve the liquid for the dipping sauce.

Filling the wrapper:

1. Preheat oven to 350 degrees. Place a small bowl of water to the side of your working space.

2. On wax paper or a clean, flat surface, lay out your egg roll wrappers.

3. Using 1 full tablespoon of mixture for each appetizer-sized wrapper, or 2 tablespoons for the larger rolls, place mixture in the center of each wrapper.

4. Top that mixture with a pinch of sprouts for each roll. Roll according to instructions on the package, rubbing some water on edge that folds over to hold roll together.

5. Lay the folded edge on baking sheet. Lightly brush each top with sesame oil.

6. Bake the rolls for 10-15 minutes until crispy. Check after 12 minutes, being cautious not to overcook.

Sesame-Ginger Dipping Sauce

Ingredients:

2 teaspoons sesame oil
1 small piece of fresh ginger, minced to equal 1 full tablespoon
1 teaspoon Tamari
Saved liquid (or gravy) from vegetable sauté
1 teaspoon toasted sesame oil
2 scallions, white and green parts, thinly sliced

Optional:
2 teaspoons agave

Procedure:

1. In a small saucepan, heat sesame oil over medium heat.
2. Add ginger and stir for 2 minutes. Add Tamari, mix well. Stir in the veggie liquid and simmer for 2 minutes.
3. Stir in the toasted sesame oil and add scallions, remove from heat immediately.
4. Stir in optional agave if you want a bit of sweetness.
5. Serve this dipping sauce at room temperature

Cook's Notes:

- Reheat your rolls in a toaster oven for 5 minutes
- The appetizer size is perfect for parties year round.
- I prefer the brand *Nasoya* for the spring roll wrappers.
- Check the *Japanese and Chinese Pantry* section in the back of the book for detailed explanations of Asian ingredients.
- If you are a vegan, read your ingredient labels to find wrappers that are egg free. Rice roll wrappers are available but they are not as soft and easy to work with as the egg roll wrapper by *Nasoya*.

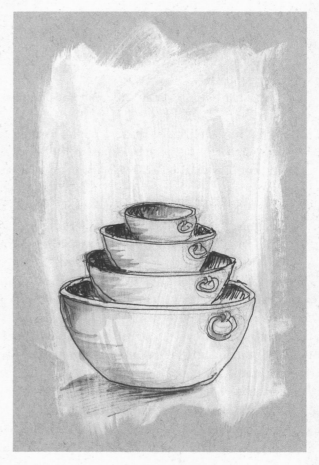

Soba-Filled Nori Rolls (Soba No Temaki)

Nori is a generic Japanese term for marine algae. Nori was first cultivated in Tokyo Bay in the seventeenth century. It has a high nutritional value because of its protein, mineral salt, and extremely high vitamin content. After the seaweed is harvested, it is washed in fresh water, dried on large frames, cut into sheets and lightly roasted. The best quality of Nori is black. A green colored variety is available in the market, and is cheaper but black is the better choice.

These vegetarian hand rolls are surprisingly delicious without raw fish. I substituted soba noodles here and delightful crunchy vegetables and watercress with just the right amount of distinctive flavor from the Umeboshi plum and wasabi powder.

Its hand crafted by you and, with some patience, can be really fun to create. Your kids can make these with you. Since Japanese cooking is very visual, your children can explore and demonstrate their creative input in this dish. Once you master the skill you can even assemble the rolls in the palm of your hands. The best part will be eating them. They have a distinctive sweet and savory taste, with a pleasing balance of flavors and textures. You can also make the rolls in an ice cream cone shape and fill with brown rice, cucumber, shrimp or salmon. What an easy way to get the kids to eat fish!

Just learning some of these authentic grocery items that are part of another culture can be exciting too. Include them in your pantry along with other healthy items from the Japanese and Chinese pantry list at the back of the book. Trying a gem of a recipe such as this one is good brain practice also, like a great crossword puzzle but this one you can eat.

They're simply creative, authentic -
Hand Rolls by your touch.

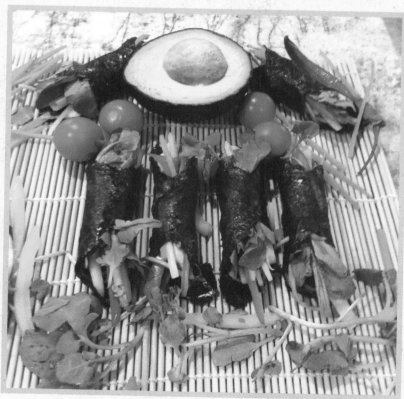

Soba-Filled Nori Rolls *(Soba No Temaki)*

Yield: 8 rolls

Ingredients:

4 ounces of uncooked Soba noodles (buckwheat pasta)
2 teaspoons sesame oil
1 tablespoon of wasabi powder
4 sheets of toasted Nori seaweed
1 avocado, peeled and thinly sliced
½ medium cucumber, deseeded and julienned,
⅛ inch by 2 inches
1 very small daikon root, peeled and julienned,
⅛ inch by 2 inches, to measure ¼ cup
½ red pepper, thinly sliced

2 tablespoons of Umeboshi paste (pickled Plum puree)
8 sprigs of fresh watercress
3 scallions, white and green parts, thinly sliced on the diagonal

Garnish:

¼ cup Tamari, for dipping
3 tablespoons of pickled ginger or 3 tablespoons of grated fresh ginger root

Procedure:

1. In a 6-quart saucepan, bring 8 cups of water to a rolling bowl. Add Soba noodles and cook for 6-8 minutes. Be cautious not to overcook. Drain and rinse in cold water, using your fingers to separate the noodles.
2. In a medium-size mixing bowl, add the noodles with two teaspoons of sesame oil. Set aside.
3. In a small prep bowl, mix 1 tablespoon of wasabi powder with 1 tablespoon and 1 teaspoon of hot water, to achieve a creamy texture. Set aside.
4. Cut each sheet of Nori in half to measure pieces 4 x 6-inches. Fill a small prep bowl of water alongside sheet for your fingertips.
5. Lay a cut Nori sheet down on a clean surface (a board or wax paper). Spread a very thin line of wasabi along the shorter edge of the Nori sheet nearest your thumb. Distribute ¼ cup of the Soba over the Nori, followed by a slice or two of the avocado, cucumber, red pepper and daikon. Sprinkle with Umeboshi paste. Place the watercress to stick out of the top of roll.
6. Place a drop of water along the edge of the bottom side of the Nori sheet, to become sticky. Roll the Nori around the filling, turning the bottom first to form a cone shape. Press the edge to stick where you put the drop of water.

7. Repeat the process for the remaining rolls. Arrange scallion pieces on top. Garnish alongside rolls with the ginger pieces or gratings and a small bowl of the Tamari.

Cook's Notes:

- This a vegetarian version of the *Temaki* hand roll. You can add a few cooked shrimp, or salmon pieces sliced thin for those who want more protein.
- The cut julienne style, is a fancy named for chopping vegetables into thin, even strips. This style is sometimes called matchstick cut. The original vegetable is divided into rectangular slices and then chopped into stick-like pieces. These matchsticks are usually ⅛ in thickness and 2 inches long. If you *Google* "how to do matchstick cut on vegetables," you can see a video which makes it easy to understand.
- I suggest *Emerald Cove Organic Pacific Nori* sheets.
- I suggest *Eden* brand for the wasabi powder and also the *Umeboshi* paste.
- Check the *Japanese and Chinese Pantry* section in the back of the book for detailed explanations of Asian ingredients.
- Have fun arranging these artistically on a special plate or as shown in the picture on a sushi roll mat, made from bamboo.

This recipe was adapted from *The Vegetarian Times Magazine 1978*.

Soba Stir-Fry (Big Noodle Bowl)

This type of noodle dish appeals to everyone, and the big bowl is visually appealing. I feel learning the art of the stir-fry is a valuable technique to master. The more you do it, the better you will become. For me, stir-frying is like a dance, have fun with it!

In French, *sauter* means to "jump". To sauté food is to make it really move over high heat, cooking it thoroughly yet quickly to retain its shape and nutritional value. Sautéing requires little time, fast action, an uncovered pan, and enough fat to coat the sauté pan. Stir-frying is just a variation of sautéing.

You have two choices here; you can use a wok, which is very professional or a sauté pan. The curved sides and rounded bottom of the wok diffuse heat and facilitate tossing and stirring. It can really be fun for the whole family to purchase a wok and the special utensils for it. However, you may have a few sauté pans as I do, and they make work fine in this application. My suggestion is to start with that option and then when you're ready, have fun exploring the different woks available.

The *Big Noodle Bowl* is a lighter fare for a fast wholesome and nutritious meal. An added bonus is the aromatics to be enjoyed after you start the sauté of the onions, garlic, ginger and scallions, and the spice ground coriander. Each adds a slightly different flavor component and depth to the dish. These fragrant plants and roots are featured in many folk remedies for common ailments. The garlic, scallions and onions belong to the botanical genus known as *Allium*. There are as many of 700 *Allium* species, and the ones I mentioned along with my favorites as, shallots, leeks, and chives are always grown for their medicinal and culinary properties, the others for decorative purposes.

This dish can be gorgeous and impressive for a dinner party or just fun for the family on a Sunday afternoon at home. You can really improvise here and be very creative with different veggies that you did not get to use during the week. It's all about sustainable ingredients that work together, like an artist's palette. Its fun cooking and the results are a *win-win* for all.

You can add your own spin to the dish with hot spices or savory spice combinations. I find it to be a dish that truly *feeds your soul*. Making it with the family extends that good feeling into the food so it serves every cell of your being. It fosters the soul to prepare and enjoy the *Big Noodle Bowl* experience together in the kitchen.

Find a special bowl to display in, with a crisp garnish and serve it with pride.

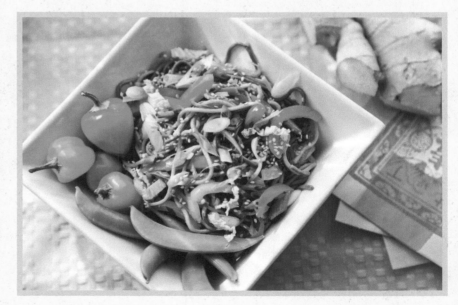

Soba Stir Fry - My Big Noodle Bowl

Yield: 6 servings

Ingredients:

1 package (8 ounces) of uncooked soba noodles (buckwheat pasta)

3 tablespoons sesame oil, divided

1 small Spanish onion, thinly sliced into half moons

6 garlic cloves, minced

2-inch knob of fresh ginger, minced to measure 2 tablespoons

6 scallions, white and green parts, thinly sliced, divided

1 teaspoon ground coriander

2 tablespoons Mirin

1½ cups thinly sliced bok choy

1 large carrot, peeled and grated

½ cup frozen edamame (shelled soybeans), rinsed

¼ cup Tamari (wheat-free soy sauce) mixed with ¼ cup water

6 medium shitake mushrooms, stems removed, thinly sliced

1 red pepper, thinly sliced

1 yellow pepper, thinly sliced

2 tablespoons of mellow white Miso paste mixed with ½ cup warm water

1½ cups snap peas, stems trimmed

2 teaspoons dark sesame oil

¼ cup chopped cilantro

Garnish:
3 tablespoons roasted sesame seeds

Procedure:

1. In a 6 to 8-quart saucepan, bring 8 cups of water to a rolling boil. Add soba noodles and boil for 6-8 minutes. Be careful not to overcook. Drain and rinse with cold water, using your fingers to separate the noodles. In a large mixing bowl add the noodles with 1 tablespoon of sesame oil, toss well to blend. Set aside.
2. In a large frying pan, skillet, or wok, sauté the onion in sesame oil until golden. Add garlic, stir 1 minute. Add ginger and half of the scallions, stirring 1 minute. Sprinkle in the coriander and mix together.
3. Increase the heat to high and add the Mirin to sizzle. Add the bok choy, carrot, and edamame, stir well.
4. Stir in the Tamari-water mixture and cover. Keep the heat up on high for 2 minutes to steam veggies.
5. Lower heat to simmer and gently add in the mushrooms, peppers and miso-water mixture. Cook for 2 minutes, keeping cover on. Add the snap peas, stir 60 seconds. Do not overcook here, keep veggies crunchy.
6. With a big spatula, fold in the above veggies with their broth, and the dark sesame oil into the soba noodles, keeping the stir-fry intact. Add the fresh cilantro.
7. Garnish with sesame seeds on top.

Cook's Notes:

- I suggest using premium organic shelled soybeans by *Cascadia Farm.*
- For the Miso Paste, I suggest using the brand *Miso Master Organic.*
- Not all soba noodles are created equal. I suggest the brand *Eden.* Their *Mugwort Soba,* is a combination of hard winter and hard spring wheat flour, whole buckwheat flour, mugwort leaf powder, and sea salt.
- There are different variations of soba noodles. Using 100% buckwheat noodles is a gluten-free option and provides a strong and heavier taste.
- Check the *Japanese and Chinese Pantry* section in the back of the book for detailed explanations of Asian ingredients.

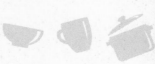

Inspired Veggie Burgers

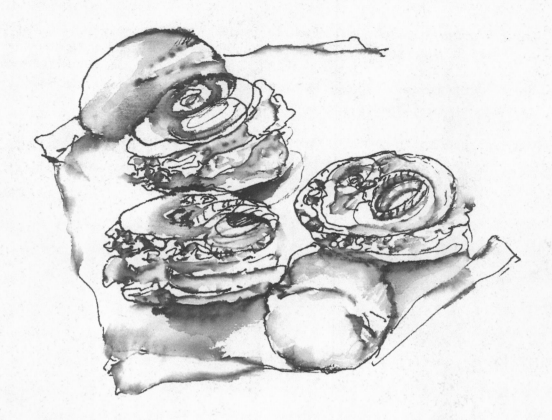

Veggie burgers are the new way of cooking healthy and fast. Most of the ingredients are simple foods with the most fundamental nutrition.

Right now, veggie burgers are appearing in the most sophisticated cookbooks and seem to cover a world of interesting ethnic tastes. I think my three recipes in this book can transform your mindset on eating less but eating better. Some people think that a veggie burger is not an adequate lunch or dinner but, on the contrary, it's a small package with giant nutrition inside.

Veggie burgers are good-for-your-heart foods. They are a smart way to create a more balanced diet as a simple and manageable way to start incorporating more beans and grains into your lifestyle. With some think ahead preparation, some of the ingredients can be prepped and ready ahead of time.

Beans have the highest vegetable source of protein. When matched up with some versatile grains, such as brown rice or quinoa, they produce a nutritional powerhouse. Most important, the burgers are more delicious than some complicated meals.

A customer I cooked for is a wonderful Yoga instructor and a busy mom of four who would have me prepare a big batch of her favorite burgers and keep them in the freezer. When she wanted them, she would simply take them out of the freezer and build them up with some suggested toppings below. She would also take them with her while traveling. Because she prefers vegan burgers, I would use ground roasted pumpkin seeds and sometimes roasted sunflower to bind them together. Burgers can be baked and not fried for the same great taste. A small amount of turmeric can be added for a brighter color without changing the taste.

Serve your burgers with a great garden salad and colorful vegetables to dramatize the burger. There's no need to flavor your burger with fatty cheese or a mainstream bun. Enjoy these suggestions for toppings: tomato salsa, horseradish spread, sweet relish, Chipotle mayo (use a non-dairy mayo, one cup with 2 teaspoons of adobe sauce to taste), grilled tomatoes, sprouts, lettuce and avocado. There are lots of choices for a better bun today, like 4-grain sprouted or a whole wheat sesame bun.

Burgers will last up to four days in the fridge. Make a big batch and turn your friends on to them. They will be grateful.

Ceci and Basmati Rice Burger

For a protein-packed Middle East feast, take the journey with me (without having to travel), to learn how to prepare this burger. I know it appeals to everyone. I have been making and serving it for years to all age groups and all taste buds. It's my friendly, easy burger. It's comforting and will truly nourish you. The brown basmati rice makes a flavorful and aromatic base for this burger.

The Italian chickpea is referred to as "ceci beans," pronounced "chech-ee." That's what we called them in my family, so this burger has roots for me. My ceci rice burgers tastes like hummus but they deliver more nutrition and that's more for your money. Hummus is the Arabic word for chickpea or garbanzo bean. It is the oldest cultivated legume, dating back 7,500 years in the Middle East. With chickpeas, you can play with the spices and tailor them to be mild or spicy.

You can tuck your burger in a pita with lettuce and tomato, avocado, cilantro, and cucumber, with a squeeze of lemon, or serve on a plate as a main dish, topped with your favorite dressing and some gorgeous chopped beets on the side. You can also break up a burger and put the pieces on top of your favorite salad instead of croutons.

I highly suggest that, just once, you make these beans from scratch. I promise that you will be hooked. If you don't have time for that, there are some great choices in your market for a better quality bean. I prefer the *Eden* brand because they cook all their beans with a piece of sea vegetable called *Kombu*.

I have great information in the "Bean Buzz" section in back of the book on the importance of using this secret ingredient to reduce any gas when eating beans. For those who are concerned with flatulence, which beans are famous for, cooking them with a small piece of the *Kombu* will most likely prevent that from happening.

As a teenager, one of my son's favorite dishes was chickpeas and pasta with lots of sautéed garlic and olive oil. Chickpeas are an essential bean in so many soups and are a favorite in many ethnic dishes. My friend Jan passed on to me a recipe that uses chickpeas, caramelized onions, and broth sautéed, then blended to make a creamy sauce over pasta. When she told me how her grown son loved it, I just had to try it. I gave it my own twist and now I cook it all the time. It's a fast dish for working moms and dads. Prepare the beans a few days ahead to make it easier.

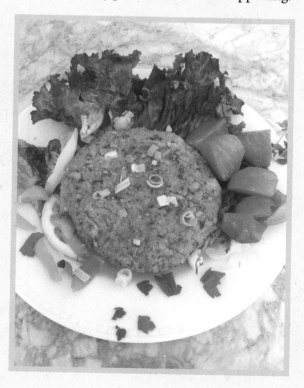

Years back when I had a café, a Rabbi who would come in to check on us because we were Kosher, told me a charming story. In the Jewish religion, at the bris of an infant boy, family and friends who have gathered to celebrate, eat when the ceremony is over (food being the centerpiece of all family occasions). Chickpeas are always served in one form or another. Because their shape is round, the child is wished a full, rounded life. Beautifully and perfectly said.

Ceci and Basmati Rice Burger

Yield: 8 burgers

Ingredients:

2 cups cooked long grain brown basmati rice (½ cup dried)
2 cups cooked garbanzo beans (1 cup dried) or 1 (15 ounce) can
¼ inch piece of Kombu seaweed, rinsed
2 tablespoons olive oil, divided
1 small red onion, medium chop
1 small Spanish onion, medium chop
4 garlic cloves, minced
1 medium jalapeno pepper, small chop
1 teaspoon ground coriander
1 teaspoon ground cumin
½ teaspoon dried thyme
Pinch of cayenne pepper
1 tablespoon Tamari (wheat-free soy sauce)
2 tablespoons Tahini (sesame paste)
1 cup grated carrots (about 1 medium-large carrot)
½ cup fresh cilantro, coarsely chopped
3 scallions, white and green parts, medium chop
2 teaspoons sea salt
¼ teaspoon ground pepper
½ cup chickpea flour or brown rice flour

Garnish:

2 tablespoons fresh lemon juice squeezed on top of each cooked and cooled burger

Optional:

2 egg whites

Procedure:

1. Preheat oven to 350 degrees. Prepare a baking sheet with natural parchment paper.
2. Rinse the rice in a tight mess strainer. In a 3 to 4-quart saucepan, bring 4 cups of water to a boil. Add rice, cover, and quickly bring to a simmer for 40 minutes. Set aside when done.
3. If using canned beans, drain and rinse with cold water to refresh. For uncooked chickpeas, soak overnight, or 5 hours in 5 cups of hot water. Rinse and drain after soaking. Throw away soaking water. For further information see the *Bean Buzz* section in back of the book.
4. In a 6 to 8-quart saucepan, bring 8 cups of water to a rolling boil. Add drained beans and Kombu. When water returns to a boil, skim off foam. Cook 40 minutes. Beans should be soft when done. Drain, discard Kombu and cool well.

5. In a medium size frying pan or saucepan, sauté the onions until soft. Stir in garlic, cook 1 minute. Add jalapeno and spices and stir to combine. Add Tamari and Tahini and stir again until well blended. Mixture may be a bit sticky here.

6. Transfer the sauté mixture to a large mixing bowl. Add the cooled beans, rice, carrots, salt and pepper, flour, chopped cilantro and scallions. Blend well and reserve ½ cup to the side.

7. In a food processor, pulse the above mixture in two batches with the reserved 1 tablespoon of oil. Do not puree the burger mixture, just pulse. You are looking for a crumbly texture. Transfer back to mixing bowl.

8. With a large spoon or ice-cream scooper, place the patties on a parchment-lined sheet tray. Using your hands (you may want to put a drop of olive oil on them) start shaping like a burger, keeping edges rounded. Leave 1 inch between burgers for flipping.

9. Cook 20 minutes. Remove from oven, wait 3 minutes and flip. Cook 6 minutes more until golden. Vegan veggie burgers can be fragile until cooked thoroughly, so flip carefully.

10. Let cool completely before storing. Wrap individually in wax paper, and place in container to store in refrigerator or freezer.

Cook's Notes:

- For time management, I suggest making more than 1 cup of beans to have on hand for another recipe during your week.
- For crispier burgers you can sauté in safflower oil using a large skillet.
- In India ground chickpea flour is called *garam besan*. You can find it today in markets such as *Fairway* and *Whole Foods*, or order online.
- *Basmati* is named after the tropical blossom of Southeast Asia.

The Healthy, Healthy Quinoa Chickpea Burger

What a dazzling duo these two nutritional giants are, handcrafted into a vegan veggie burger. A powerful duo like Batman and Robin! Quinoa and chickpeas are the perfect combination for a kick-start breakfast or a high-fiber lunch.

Chickpeas, also known as garbanzo beans, are called the *king bean* because they contain more iron than any other bean. Chickpeas, as well as quinoa, have seeds that are coated with *Saponins*. They have compounds in the plant that can fight off insects and the effects of pesticides, a built-in pest detergent. Thus, they supply much endurance and strength in your body. Research studies indicate that diets rich in *Saponins* reduce the plasma cholesterol by 12 percent to 24 percent.

Because of their high protein content, beans are body-building warming foods. They provide us with the protein needed for body repair without saddling us with cholesterol, fat, and toxic nitrogen by-products of meat. Also, the grain has a high-fiber content. Diets high in fiber are associated with reduced risk of colorectal cancer.

Quinoa's claim to fame is its high amino acid protein content. The United Nations Food and Agricultural Organization states that quinoa is closer to the ideal protein balance than any other common grain, being at least equal to milk in protein quality. While no single food can supply all of the essential life-sustaining nutrients, quinoa comes as close as any other in the vegetable or animal kingdom. It has earned the phrase "mother of all grains" for that reason. Quinoa is remarkably high in B vitamins, iron, and zinc. Its thiamine content is higher than that of chicken liver, which is considered the superior B source. Quinoa is easy to digest because it contains no gluten. Quinoa is a valuable part of a vegetarian diet.

Be creative with this grain: purée with fruit for baby food; purée cooked quinoa into hummus; for a supercharged breakfast, cook with oats, cinnamon, amaranth, and raisins. It makes a great Greek pie, baked with feta, dill, and eggs.

To come up with a great burger, practice makes perfect. It takes no time at all before you get the hang of it, as they say. Try making them with a friend and sharing the burgers. I am all for "buddy cooking" (cooking with a friend who has the same philosophies as you do about health) and then you have some company and have a goal to reach together. Whether you are a meat-eater, vegan, vegetarian or flexitarian, burgers will fit into your lifestyle perfectly and effortlessly. This grain/bean duo should be an essential part of your diet.

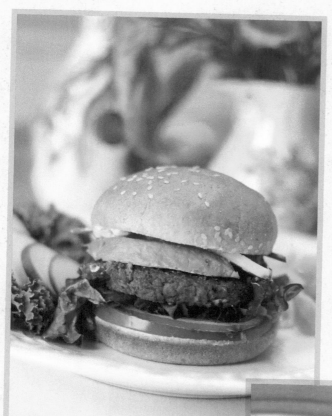

Quinoa Chickpea Burger

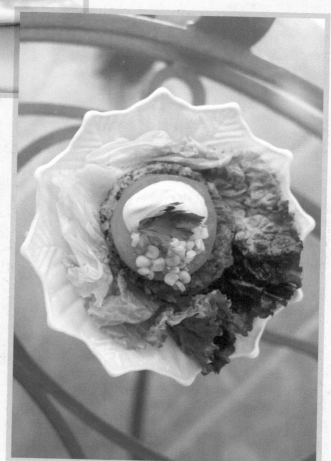

Sweet Sonny Burger

Quinoa Chickpea Burger

Yield: 8 burgers

Ingredient:

1 ½ cups cooked quinoa
1 medium yam or sweet potato, cooked and mashed
1 -15 ounce and ½ cans of Garbanzo beans
    (chickpeas)
1 cup walnuts, roasted, small chop
1 tablespoon olive oil
1 small red onion, medium chop
1 small Spanish onion, medium chop
6 cloves of garlic, minced
1 tablespoon jalapeno pepper, small chop
1 teaspoon ground coriander
1 teaspoon oregano
1 teaspoon ground paprika
½ teaspoon cumin

½ teaspoon chipotle pepper
1 carrot, small chop
2 celery stalks, small chop
1 tablespoon Tamari (wheat-free soy sauce)
2 teaspoons sea salt
2 teaspoons fresh lemon juice
¼ teaspoon ground pepper
½ cup cilantro, coarsely chop
¼ cup Italian flat-leaf parsley, coarsely chop
2 tablespoons dairy-free mayonnaise, such as
    Vegenaise
3 scallions, white and green parts, medium chop
½ red pepper, small chop
½ yellow pepper, small chop

Optional:

2 teaspoons sesame oil

Procedure:

Prepare a baking sheet with natural parchment paper
Preheat oven at any point to 350 degrees

1. Cook 1 cup quinoa by, soaking the grain 1-2 minutes. Rinse through a tight mess strainer. Bring 1 ¾ cups water to a boil, add grain, lower to a simmer for 23 minutes, and then cool before using. Scoop out 1 ½ cups for the burgers, set aside.
2. Steam or bake sweet potato, set aside to cool. Steaming is a fast procedure, peel and medium chop, steam for 7-8 minutes in a steamer basket or until soft.
3. Drain and rinse beans in strainer and set aside to dry in strainer, stir frequently.
4. Roast walnuts at 350 degrees for 6 minutes, cool and chop.
5. In a medium size frying pan or saucepan, sauté the 2 onions in olive oil until soft, stir in garlic, cook 1 minute, add jalapeno, and all above spices, stir until blended. Add Tamari, carrots and celery and cook until soft not mushy.
6. In a big large mixing bowl, blend cooled grain, beans, the sauté, fresh herbs, salt and pepper.
7. In a food processor start to pulse most of the mixture with the mayo leaving aside one full cup. If it is a small machine do in two batches. You need to look for a crumbly texture here. Return to the big bowl and stir in walnuts, raw peppers, scallions and lemon juice and then fold in the reserved one cup of mixture. If the mixture is on the drier side you can add the sesame oil here by eye.

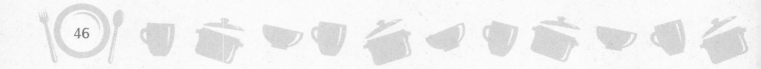

8. With a big spoon or large ice-cream scooper, place patties on sheet tray, then with your hands (you may want to put a drop of olive oil on them) start shaping like a hamburger.

9. Bake 20 minutes, remove from oven, let them rest 5 minutes, then turn carefully with an oiled spatula onto your hand and then slide unto pan. (Vegan veggie burgers can be fragile until cooked thoroughly). Cook burgers 6 minutes more until firm and crispy.

10. Let cool on tray before storing. Wrap individual burgers in wax paper when cooled, then place in container to store in refrigerator or freezer.

Cook's Notes:

- The cooked quinoa will yield more than you need, so use the rest in egg scrambles, wraps, bean salads or my favorite, pancakes. (Never make less than a cup of this Supergrain)
- These are vegan burgers, you can use eggs, and I suggest egg whites. Omit the mayo, and use 2 whites in mixture putting in while food processors are running.
- Top your burgers with cheddar cheese, avocado, lettuce and tomato.
- Burgers will stay fresh up to 4-5 days depending on you refrigerator.

Sweet Sonny Burger

My daughter, who is an amazing working mom, asked me to come up with a healthy burger for her son, one that she could freeze and use for dinners or lunch. The baby was around 15 months old and really showing signs at that age of being a young vegetarian.

One of his very first meals, after fruits and veggies, was mushy red lentils and brown rice, made by his mom. He loved it. He definitely felt her love in that dish. A child has to be a good chewer, because a bean may be difficult to digest until they are older. A child should not have a bean everyday at a young age. Rotation of food is very important for them, as it is for everyone.

Creating a veggie burger can be a challenge. They need to have some essentials such as: a bean or bean combination for protein; a whole grain such as brown rice, millet or quinoa; onions or garlic for flavor; flavorful spices; pungent flavors, zesty or nutty; herbs for freshness; eggs or mayo for binding. You can create one with this formula, but it's important to know who you are creating it for and what are their nutritional needs.

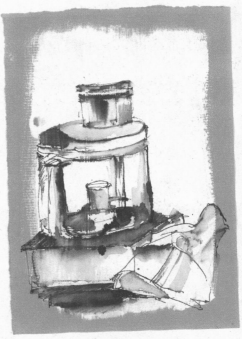

The Food Processor-your useful tool for making veggie burgers

If you're a newcomer to all this, I suggest starting with the black bean (also called black turtle beans). They are very easy to digest, are a blood tonic and fall under an alkalizing food (which is wonderful for balance because most American foods are acid forming). They have a sweet flavor which, when combined with brown rice make a perfect marriage.

I encourage you not to use canned beans here. Don't cheat your loved ones out of the authentic taste of home cooked black beans. Cook up a batch from scratch and give it your best shot. It will be your head start for serving nutritionally rich foods. Beans build energy and are heart smart foods.

So our little guy is now eating a burger with high protein, vitamins and minerals and anti-oxidants. Coconut oil, cooked in the rice provides a good source of omega-3. It's a pretty looking burger too! We broke up the burger into small pieces, which was appropriate for his size. He now loves avocado so that will always be a nutritious garnish on his burger.

This is also a great burger for fussy teenagers who have a lack of protein in their diet. You can choose a sharper cheddar cheese and then make the burger inviting and fun by wrapping it in a burrito topped with a juicy tomato, red onion, ketchup and soft lettuce. This burger may just end up being your favorite burger. Make a double batch and share with loved ones.

Sweet Sonny Burger

Yield: 8 regular burgers or 14 slider size

Ingredients:

1 cup uncooked organic black beans
¼ inch piece of Kombu seaweed, rinsed
2 cups cooked medium brown basmati rice (1 cup uncooked)
1 teaspoon organic virgin coconut oil
1 medium yam or sweet potato, peeled, cooked, and mashed
½ sweet yellow onion, peeled, small chop
2 tablespoons olive oil, divided
5-6 ounces of hormone-free sharp cheddar cheese, grated
¼ cup cilantro, coarsely chopped
¼ cup Italian flat-leaf parsley, coarsely chopped
2 teaspoons sea salt
¼ teaspoon freshly ground black pepper
1 large organic whole egg plus one egg white
2-3 tablespoons safflower or grape seed oil (for the grill)

Procedure:

1. Sort out the beans for small rocks or dirt. Spread out on a white plate or cutting board for a clearer vision.
2. Soak overnight or for 5 hours in hot water. Rinse and drain after soaking. Throw away soaking water. (For further information see the "Bean Buzz" section in back of book).
3. In a 6 to 8-quart saucepan, bring 7 cups of water to a rolling boil. Add drained beans and Kombu. When water returns to a boil, skim off foam. Cook 40 minutes. Beans should be soft, not mushy, when done. Drain, save softened Kombu with the beans, and cool well.
4. Rinse the rice in a tight mess strainer. In a 4-6 quart saucepan, bring 2 cups of water to a boil. Add rinsed rice and the coconut oil. Stir and lower to a slow simmer for 40 minutes, covered. During the cooking process stir one to two times. You are creating a "stickier" rice for the burger. When rice is done, measure out 2 cups needed for the recipe. Allow rice to cool. Save the rest for another meal.
5. Steam or bake sweet potato, set aside to cool. Steaming is a simple procedure: peel and medium chop your potatoes, steam for 7-8 minutes in a steamer basket, or until soft
6. In a small frying pan, sauté the onion until soft and golden.
7. Grate the cheese by hand against the largest hole of a stand-up grater.
8. Preheat the grill to 400 degrees, or a skillet to medium-high.
9. In a small cup whisk together the egg and egg white.
10. In a large mixing bowl add cooled rice, beans, fresh herbs, salt and pepper, mashed sweet potato, and the eggs. Blend well using a rubber spatula. Stir in grated cheese. Reserve one cup of the mixture.
11. In a food processor pulse the mixture into a smooth texture. If the machine is small, work in two batches. Put mixture back into the mixing bowl with the reserved cup and blend well to incorporate. Your burger will have tiny pieces of black beans and rice.

12. Scoop desired amount of mixture with a large spoon or ice cream scooper and place on a flat surface covered with wax paper. With your hands or the back of a spoon, shape into burgers or sliders.

13. Using a brush or back of a wooden spoon, spread 2-3 tablespoons of oil on the grill. Place burgers down leaving a ½ inch space between them for easy flipping (see photo). Cook for 5 minutes and then lower heat to 350 degrees.

14. Flip and cook for 8 to 10 minutes until crispy. Depending on the surface of your grill or skillet, you may have to flip 3 times to get desired crispiness without burning. Cool on rack for 10 minutes.

Cook's Notes:

- As explained in the forward to this recipe, cook the beans from scratch for an authentic flavor. From a culinary and nutritional viewpoint the taste is definitely better and the nutritional content much greater.
- By all means cook more rice if you prefer more than one cup. To serve a family with this recipe for the week, one cup of basmati rice yields 3 ⅓ cups rice. Get creative, use left-over rice for stir-fry's or under steamed vegetables.
- Rice is also known as "the bread of half the world."
- You can also bake the burgers in the oven on a sheet pan with parchment paper. If you do this, do not oil the paper. Bake 20 minutes, flip, and continue baking for another 6 minutes.
- When re-heating, add a small amount of grated cheddar cheese on top along with a juicy tomato.

Versatile Vegetarian Sides

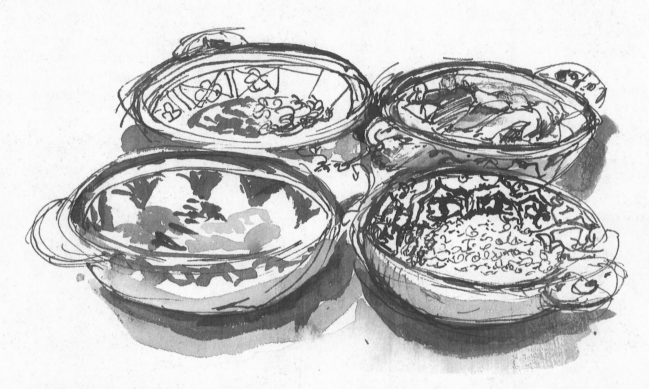

There are hundreds of varieties of legumes which provide a primary source of protein for millions of vegetarians all around the world. Experts often describe legumes as excellent "nutritional bargains." Not only do they cost less than meat but they are good sources of protein, fiber, iron, several B vitamins, potassium and magnesium and have very little fat. Legumes are also rich in folate, a B-vitamin that protects people against heart attacks and other coronary illnesses by lowering blood levels of homocysteine, an amino acid associated with an increased heart disease rate. Research suggests that 400 micrograms of folate is sufficient to keep homocysteine levels down in most adults. This amount of folate equals a cup of cooked lentils, black eye peas, or chickpeas.

The two following recipes in this chapter are really thinking out-of-the-box if you're basically eating an "All American Diet." I can wholeheartedly say to you that learning about new food groups and their cultural spices are a great discovery and changing your diet can truly change your life.

Chickpeas are part of a spectacular group of foods that are called *Hydrophilic* foods, or *water-loving foods*. They are foods loaded with soluble fiber. They keep us feeling fuller longer, which help with weight loss, diminish cravings and aid in maintaining digestive health. They contain an appetite- regulating hormone called ghrelin. Some other examples of *Hydrophilic* foods that you've been hearing a lot of nutritional news on are; chia seeds, red kidney beans, oatmeal, and Brussel sprouts.

I talk so much about chickpeas and other legumes in my book because I feel if you're a newcomer to some of these healthier recipes, these two are heart-smart, accessible foods to include in your action plan right away.

I encourage parents to tell stories about the origins of these simple, yet nutrient-rich foods. You will surely captivate your children's minds with facts for them to remember as they go through their life's journey. My grown children are still reminding me of all the stories told at the dinner table (and then they laugh at me), but now that they are cooking for their family dinners, memories come back and they are enjoying cooking from these food groups that they know are so good for them. In my café we always included food stories and facts on the bulletin board and I saw people really enjoyed reading them and asking questions, which I loved to see.

A note of history on the chickpea, it is said to have been first cultivated about 5000 AD in ancient Mesopotamia, then moved to the eastern Mediterranean and into India and other parts of Asia. The chickpeas were introduced to Spain where it was (and is) called garbanzos. Peci is its Italian name.

So get excited; don't just open a can of beans or legumes (a lot less sodium if you don't). It's worth the effort it takes to soak dried beans or legumes overnight on a Friday or Saturday, and then cook them up on Sunday while you're home getting things done for the week and just resting. You'll love the aroma from the pot, with just a bay leaf and some garlic.

It will be a great start to your meatless monday, trying my tender, creamy, flavor-packed Chana Saag, and the 3-Way Bounty Butternut Casserole.

The Perfect Zen Combo- All in One Pot Meal

While working for a publishing company in the mid-80s, I sat at a desk for long periods of time. I needed to bring to work a well-rounded nutritious dish to eat anytime I could fit it in--breakfast, lunch, or dinner. I created this all-in-one-pot dish that can stay out of refrigeration for about 8 hours. It was a lifesaver for me when I worked crazy hours! Even better, it's a delicious combination of foods that equal *nourishing goodness*.

Organic brown rice has been part of Zen bowls from the beginning of time, calming to the nerves with its high protein count. Butternut, a winter squash, now available six months out of the year, was used extensively by early American settlers. Pilgrims adopted this versatile vegetable as its own. It is part of the *cucurbita* family, which includes hard-skinned and tender-skinned squash. Besides being both sweet and savory in flavor (especially with the addition of herbs and spices as sage, rosemary and cinnamon) butternut squash is a rich source of beta-carotene, powerful antioxidants, and anti-inflammatory properties.

The lentils in this dish melt into the softened rice and give the pot another blast of protein. Lentils date back to Biblical times. They have been a staple food in the Middle East for thousands of years. A cup of cooked lentils packs a gram more protein then a 3-ounce patty of lean ground meat. Wow!

Arame, a popular mild sea vegetable has superior nutritional content. It's infused in this dish at the end. Sea vegetables transmit the energies of the sea to the body as a rich source of protein, complex carbohydrates, minerals, and vitamins. They provide a full-spectrum concentration of beta-carotene, chlorophyll, enzymes, amino acids, and fiber. Their distinctive salty taste is not just salt, but a balanced combination of sodium, potassium, calcium, magnesium, phosphorus, iron, and trace minerals. Arame converts these ocean minerals into organic mineral salts that combine with amino acids. Our bodies can use this combination as an ideal way to get usable nutrients for structural building blocks. Sea vegetables are almost the only non-animal source of Vitamin B-12 necessary for cell development and nerve function. Their mineral balance builds sound nerve structure, and proper metabolism and this is a relaxing effect on mind and body. To finish off the Zen pot are precious "cran-jewels," that which have natural benefits beyond basic nutrition. Cranberries have antibacterial properties which account for their "superstar status." In Colonial times, cranberries were believed to be medicine; and they were called a symbol of peace but most importantly were used as a functional food.

Other cultures around the world have their authentic variation of this dish. In Italy (my grandparents' roots) the version of this dish, or one pot meal, is called *cucina provera*. There is no adequate translation, though *"the poor cook"* or *"country food"* reflects the dish. Italians treat their food as an extension of the way they live, surrounded by family and the people they love. The ingredients are seasonal and therefore, the best in quality and price, and the preparation is easy. Many star chefs promote this style of cooking today.

3-Way Bounty Butternut Casserole

Yield 6 servings

Ingredients:

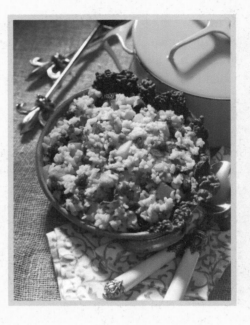

1 cup short grain brown rice
3 cups water, ½ reserved
2 teaspoons organic virgin coconut oil or raw coconut butter
1 teaspoon sea salt
¼ cup green or brown lentils
1 small butternut squash, peeled and cut into ¼ inch chunks, about
    2 cups measured
1 tablespoon Arame seaweed, soaked in water for 8 minutes
¼ cup and 1 tablespoon dried unsweetened cranberries, rinsed

Optional:
2 teaspoons of butter or ghee (clarified butter)

Procedure:

1. Rinse the rice in a tight mesh strainer. In a 4-6 quart sauce pan, bring 2½ cups water to boil. Add rinsed rice and coconut oil. Stir and lower to a simmer for 20 minutes with cover.
2. After twenty minutes, bring the water back up to boil, with the ½ cup reserved water and lentils, butternut, and sea salt
3. Let mixture boil for 12 minutes, until butternut is soft but not mushy. You may have to add a tablespoon or two of water if it looks like water is evaporating too quickly.
4. Rinse and soak the Arame for 8 minutes, then rinse and drain and chop coarsely.
5. Drop the seaweed into the pot, (it will be almost the end of cooking time for rice, butternut, lentil mixture, stir in the cranberries, blend well and cook for 5 minutes more on simmer.
6. Adjust the sea salt. Add butter or ghee at end.

Cook's Notes:

- A nourishing meal for breakfast, lunch or dinner
- Get ahead and prep the butternut the day before
- The Arame seaweed is tricky to measure exactly, so fill up a tablespoon and it will work. I suggest *Eden* brand it is wild and hand harvested
- I suggest only organic for the butternut, non-organic tastes flat

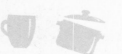

Aromatic Chana Saag

Indian food has a special flare, with its heart and soul revealed in its unique spice combinations. It's fun discovering and learning the distinctive spices of India. I suppose many of you probably are familiar with such spices as cinnamon, ginger coriander, cumin, and cloves. A number of India's favorite flavorings are also notable for their health-promoting properties.

Part of my joy in cooking is when flavors and aromas start to come together. It's just that way in the preparation of this dish. Chana Saag is a very quick dish to assemble; it will probably become a favorite of yours. When you can find strong, dark green perky spinach, it's the time to make this dish. Of course you can use baby spinach in the bag if you can't find the thicker, darker Popeye spinach which is much richer in taste.

Chickpeas, the king bean, should always be in your pantry. Soaking these beans will surely make them digestible and delicious. Make sure you make a double batch to prepare some homemade hummus or roast some in the oven for an after school snack for the children. These two combinations, beans and spinach, are the fundamental nutrients here. Vitamins, minerals and antioxidants from all the herbs are the bonus. You can make it as spicy as you like; know who you're serving it to.

A client I had for many years would frequent a famous Indian restaurant in New York City and enjoyed ordering this dish from time to time. He asked me if I could copy it. So I did a search on the Internet and found about 6 versions of the recipe. I ended up combining them and, with fresh spinach and great pureed tomatoes imported from Italy, started to make the dish. When I was sautéing the ginger, garlic and jalapeno pepper mixed with the special spices, I knew then the tantalizing flavors would make this a great dish. The home cooked chickpeas combined with the tomato and herbs, lots of fresh cilantro, and finished off with organic coconut milk was a great cultural event, that day.

I was not exposed to this type of cooking growing up, but since the global market exploded, these ingredients are found everywhere. I have been making it for friends and family ever since. Serve it right from the pot; it looks so soulful at its spicy, healthy best.

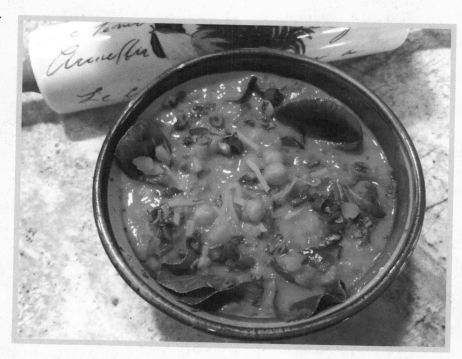

Aromatic Chana Saag (Chickpeas with Spinach)

Yield: 6-8 servings

Ingredients:

1 cup uncooked chickpeas or 2 (15 ounce) cans, drained and rinsed
¼ inch piece of Kombu seaweed, rinsed
2 tablespoons olive oil
1 Spanish onion, medium chop
4 large garlic cloves or 6 medium, minced
½-inch piece ginger root, minced to measure 1 tablespoon
1 jalapeno pepper, deseeded and minced
1 (14.5 ounce) can of crushed tomatoes
1 (12-14 ounce) can of coconut milk
1 pound fresh spinach, washed, medium chop
2 tablespoons fresh lemon juice
½ cup cilantro, finely chopped
2 teaspoons sea salt
¼ teaspoon freshly ground pepper

Spices:

2 teaspoons ground coriander
1 teaspoon ground cumin
1 teaspoon curry powder
1 teaspoon ground turmeric
½ teaspoon red chili powder
¼ teaspoon ground cinnamon
¼ teaspoon ground cardamom
¼ teaspoon ground cloves
¼ teaspoon cayenne pepper

Garnish:

6 plum tomatoes, deseeded, small chop

Procedure:

1. If using canned beans, drain and rinse with cold water to refresh. For uncooked chickpeas, soak overnight, or 5 hours in 5 cups of hot water. Rinse and drain after soaking. Throw away soaking water. For further information see the *Bean Buzz* section in the back of the book.
2. In a 6 to 8-quart saucepan, bring 8 cups water to a rolling boil. Add drained beans and Kombu. When water returns to a boil, skim off foam. Cook for 40 minutes. Beans should be firm and hold their shape. Drain, reserving ½ cup of the cooking liquid.
3. In a large-size saucepan pan, sauté the onion in olive oil until golden. Add garlic and ginger and stir for 1 minute. Add jalapeno pepper, cooking 1 minute more.

4. In a small prep bowl, measure out the aromatic spices. Add to the sauté with the cayenne pepper and stir to blend well.
5. Add cooked chickpeas with the ½ cup reserved cooking liquid, or ½ cup water if using canned beans. Bring to a low boil. Add tomatoes and salt, cook for 10 minutes.
6. Stir in the coconut milk, lower heat and cook 5 minutes.
7. Gently fold in the spinach, cover, and allow to wilt for 3 minutes. Add lemon juice, cilantro, and pepper. Taste and adjust salt.
8. Garnish with fresh plum tomatoes.

Cook's Notes:

* This recipe uses a sultry spice combo. If you don't have all the spices on hand, you can substitute 2 teaspoons of *garam masala*.
* *Garam masala* is a blend of fragrant ground spices common in North Indian and other Asian cuisines. It can be used alone or with other spices. The word "garam" refers to the intensity of spices.
* For a heartier Chana Saag, add brown rice and cooked cauliflower.
* Depending on where you live, dark colored spinach with the thicker leaves may not available all year. You can use Swiss chard if fresh spinach is not in season.
* Check the *Bean Buzz* section of the book to read more about cooking beans from scratch.

Good morning, Breakfast!

Breakfast is the cornerstone of today's health-conscious cuisine. It should set the stage for a vigorous day of sustained energy. I never miss breakfast. I consider it a sacred meal. Breakfast is breaking an overnight fast so I suggest taking your time to figure out what type of breakfast can nourish you well. My most productive and fulfilling days start with a power breakfast (or a protein smoothie.)

If you're a mom or dad raising a family, it is important to know that young children's growing demands certainly require a hearty breakfast. There are numerous clinical studies that show that it is key for students to eat a nutritious breakfast for their attention span and improved grades. These students also have fewer sick days. Isn't it a great honor to establish good breakfast habits for your children to have for a lifetime? Don't they deserve this?

Those of us with the luxury of time can have enhanced breakfast rituals that are usually associated with Sunday morning, holidays, or a vacation morning. I like to teach parents that a weekday breakfast can be just as creative and delicious as those rituals. It requires good time management skills in your weekly menu planning and shopping. Aim to be more organized in the kitchen. An example of that might be washing and chopping fresh fruits and vegetables ahead of time, measuring out ingredients.

In our Power Pancake recipe, I cook the grain the day before, and measure out the dry ingredients. I make a big batch so I have extra for my freezer pantry. However, I never store it for more than two weeks. (We eat the pancakes too fast.) I am confident that, even frozen, these pancakes are a great choice, packed with whole grain goodness, protein, and berry power (blueberries are high in antioxidants). If you don't want to top with syrup, make some poached or sautéed apples or pears for that special touch. Remember that whole grains such as quinoa (pronounced "keen-wa") nourished the world's greatest ancient civilizations. The super grain evokes energy and good health, a great way to start the day.

Create some kitchen magic with my Farm–to-Table Frittata. Eggs contain essential nutrients. They are easily digested and their protein almost fully utilized by the body. (I prefer organic whole eggs, the yolks and whites are a great source of Vitamin D.) In this dish, eggs are whirled around with all these delicious vegetables, in a pie-like form. It can go from breakfast to lunch or a light dinner with a great salad. This can be made Sunday night and warmed up.

Breakfast muffins are part of the "grab and go culture" of today. My Spiced Carrot Bran Muffins have won the hearts of some friends and customers who have certain constipation issues. The unprocessed bran adds a rich source of valuable fiber to your diet. The fresh carrots boast an important shot of beta carotene. But don't be fooled; it tastes more like a dessert muffin. The carrots, raisins, molasses, maple, and flavorful spices all contribute to its special status.

Breakfast foods are as diverse as the people in the world. It is so interesting to me to learn about the culinary customs of international breakfasts around the world. You can be inspired by them too. Share the knowledge and enthusiasm with your family. Create some magic at breakfast time. If not during the week, weekends can be a start for some new ideas.

Quinoa Power Pancakes

Yield: 6 servings

My two children and husband named these pancakes "Power Pancakes" because you can literally go all day without being hungry and have optimum energy. You can be creative also combining different flour combinations with other berries and nuts.

Ingredients:

1 cup uncooked quinoa
½ cup quinoa flour
½ cup yellow cornmeal
½ cup rolled oats
1 tablespoon ground flax seed
1 tablespoon chia seeds
¾ cup walnuts, small chop
1 tablespoon natural dry sugar
1 teaspoon non-aluminum baking powder

½ teaspoon baking soda
½ teaspoon sea salt
1 whole egg plus 1 egg white
1 cup low-fat buttermilk, or plain yogurt
3 tablespoons melted organic butter
3 tablespoons of *Earth Balance* organic buttery
   spread, divided
½ cup fresh blueberries, or frozen (if frozen thaw
   and drain before using)

Spices:

1½ teaspoon ground cinnamon
½ teaspoon ground ginger
¼ teaspoon ground nutmeg
¼ teaspoon ground cardamom

Garnish:

Fresh pears or peaches according to season

Procedure:

1. Cook quinoa by soaking grain 1-2 minutes. Rinse through a tight mess strainer. Bring 1 ¾ cups water to a boil, add grain, lower to a simmer for 23 minutes, and then cool before using. Measure out one cup cooked for pancakes. Set aside the rest (see cooks notes).
2. Preheat griddle to 375-400 degrees. Depending on the pan, degrees may vary.
3. In a medium-size bowl, measure out and mix together all dry ingredients and spices. Fold in cooked, cooled quinoa.
4. Melt butter over low heat, be careful not to burn.
5. Whisk together egg and egg white, buttermilk, and the melted butter.
6. Blend the wet with the dry ingredients until well blended, don't over mix.
7. Stir in blueberries with soft spatula, being careful not to break berries.
8. Grease pan with *Earth Balance*, spread well.
9. On the prepared griddle, ladle ¼ cup of batter to form a pancake. After about 4 minutes, when pancakes are puffy and a few bubbles form, flip carefully to the other side. Give them another 3 minutes on that side. After second batch re-grease the pan.

Cook's Notes:

- Quinoa can be made a day or two before for good time management. One cup of quinoa relates to: 8g of protein; 5g of fiber 15% DV iron, plus heart healthy omega 3 fatty acids.
- The quinoa will yield more than you need for the pancakes, so use the rest in a great pilaf or soup, or scramble with eggs and use in a wrap with other cooked veggies.
- For the natural sugar in this recipe, I used dark coconut sugar.
- Try these natural alternatives to white sugar; blonde or dark coconut sugar; date sugar; sucanat; organic granulated sugar; xylitol; stevia (this one is very strong, use in baking replace one cup sugar with one teaspoon stevia powder). All of these are found in markets as; *Whole Foods* and *Fairway*. Many can also be purchased on line.
- You can purchase quinoa flour as well as other quinoa products by going to Google and typing in, *Ancient Harvest* products.
- When pancakes cool, wrap them in wax paper to store in refrigerator or freezer.

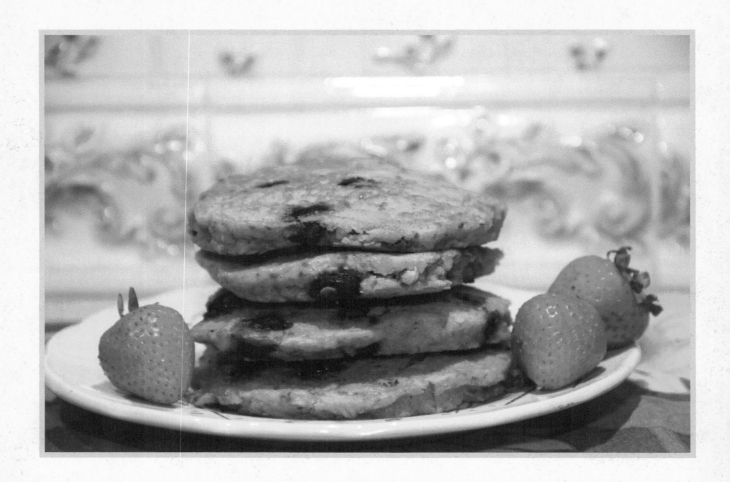

Farm to Table - Asparagus, Leek and Potato Frittata

Yield: 4-6 servings

Ingredients:

6 asparagus stalks, steamed and cut into ⅛-inch pieces
4 small baby red potatoes, cooked 10 minutes, thinly sliced
2 tablespoons olive oil
¼ medium Spanish onion, small chop
1 large leek, white part only, small chop
½ teaspoon dried thyme
2 plum tomatoes, deseeded, small chop
½ red pepper, small chop
6 organic eggs
1 tablespoon freshly grated Parmesan cheese
2 tablespoons Italian flat-leaf parsley, small chop, divided
2 tablespoons fresh chives, small chop, divided
1 teaspoon sea salt
¼ teaspoon freshly ground pepper
2 teaspoons butter

Optional:

1 tablespoon fresh basil to add to above herbs (when available)
2 cups fresh arugula or spinach as a base for the plate

Procedure:

1. Snap (or cut) off woody ends of the asparagus. In a steamer basket add asparagus stalks to steam 2 minutes. Remove, cool 1 minute, and cut into ⅛-inch pieces. Set aside.
2. In a 6 to 9-quart saucepan, bring 6 cups of cold water and potatoes to a boil. Cook for 10 minutes, you want them to be firm. Drain, cool (you can put in the refrigerator for 10 minutes), slice very thin (almost like paper) keeping red skins intact, set aside.
3. In an 8-inch skillet or saucepan, sauté onion in olive oil until golden. Stir in the leek and cook for 2 minutes until soft. Stir in the thyme, asparagus, tomatoes, and red pepper. Cook for 1 minute. Transfer this sauté to a small bowl. Wipe the pan out with a paper towel and set pan aside.
4. In a medium-size bowl, whisk eggs with Parmesan cheese, parsley, chives, salt, and pepper. Add the above sauté and fold in to combine.
5. In the preheated pan, melt the butter with 1 tablespoon of oil, swirling around, making sure sides are greased. Immediately pour the egg mixture with the veggies into pan (you want the pan hot). Gently stir to distribute the vegetables, letting the eggs set a bit, about 2 minutes. Reduce heat to low and cook 4 minutes. The sides should begin to look golden.
6. In a circular design place sliced red potatoes on top just to fit the pan.
7. Preheat the broiler of a toaster oven, or regular oven, to high.

8. Place the pan under heat and broil until the top of the frittata is puffed out and golden brown, about 3-4 minutes. If the top begins to get to brown, cover with foil. Reduce oven temperature to 375 degrees. Be careful here, the handle will be very hot. Cook frittata for 5 minutes.
9. The frittata is done when top is firm. To serve loosen the frittata by running a thin spatula along the sides. Slide frittata onto a platter. Cut into wedges. Garnish with addition chives, parsley, and basil.

Cook's Notes:

- If baby red potatoes are not available small Yukon potatoes will do.
- I like to keep a non-stick enamel pan with a handle that is ovenproof in my inventory for this recipe.
- To cut cooking time, prep the veggies the day before and put into a tightly sealed container.
- As mentioned in the forward, Frittata's make the best leftovers the next day. Place over a salad or enjoy on its own. Bon Appetite!

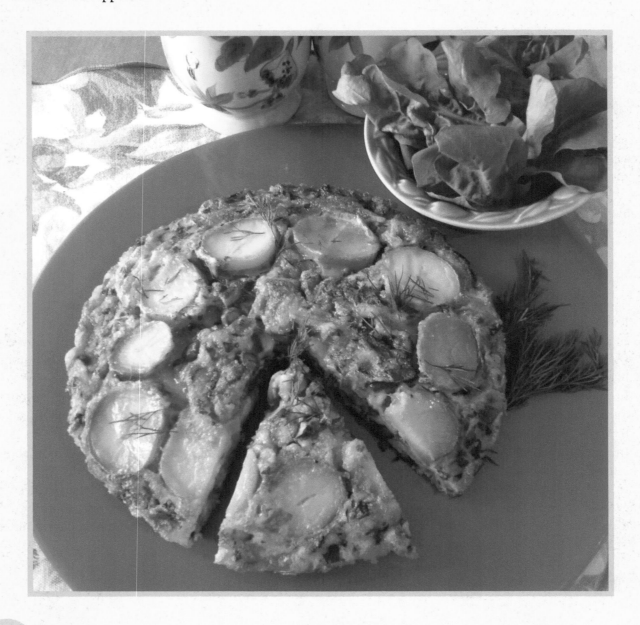

Spiced Carrot Bran Muffins

Yield: 25-30 muffins

Dry Ingredients:

1½ cups spelt flour
1½ cups barley flour
3 cups coarse bran, also known as Miller's Bran
1 teaspoon sea salt
2 teaspoons baking soda
2 teaspoons non-aluminum baking powder

Spices:

1½ teaspoons ground cinnamon
¼ teaspoon ground cardamom
¼ teaspoon ground nutmeg
¼ teaspoon ground allspice
⅛ teaspoon ground cloves

Wet Ingredients:

4 large egg whites
2½ cups almond, rice or soy milk
¼ cup safflower or grape seed oil
1 cup grade B maple syrup or ⅔ cup honey
½ cup molasses

4 tablespoons apple cider vinegar
2 teaspoons pure vanilla extract
2 cups carrots (about 3 carrots), peeled and grated
1½ cup organic raisins

Procedure:

1. Preheat oven to 375 degrees. Oil muffin pans or use unbleached baking cups (do not oil baking cups).
2. In a large bowl, mix dry ingredients with the spices.
3. In a small bowl, whisk egg whites.
4. In a medium bowl blend all wet ingredients.
5. Mix the wet into the dry ingredients alternately with the carrots and the raisins. Let this mixture sit for 10-15 minutes.
6. Fill muffin cups ¾ full.
7. Bake 20 minutes or until muffin bounces back to touch. Cool on rack before wrapping.

Cook's Notes:

- As long as the yield equals 3 cups of flour, you can use other flour combinations for this recipe. For example: sprouted whole wheat, rye, brown rice, millet, quinoa, and buckwheat.
- *Shiloh Farms* makes an excellent coarse bran sold in all health food stores. You can also find it at *Whole Foods* and *Fairway* markets, and online.
- This mixture can stay in the refrigerator for up to two days. Bring to room temperature before baking. Cooked muffins stay fresh for 4 days.
- The muffins freeze well, hence the reason for the large yield. My past experience with customers proved this to be true, as well as dear friends who make these muffins all the time for their families.
- Molasses is an excellent source of potassium, calcium and iron.
- Fiber is a major component in a healthy diet. Make this "anytime" muffin a part of your healthier lifestyle.

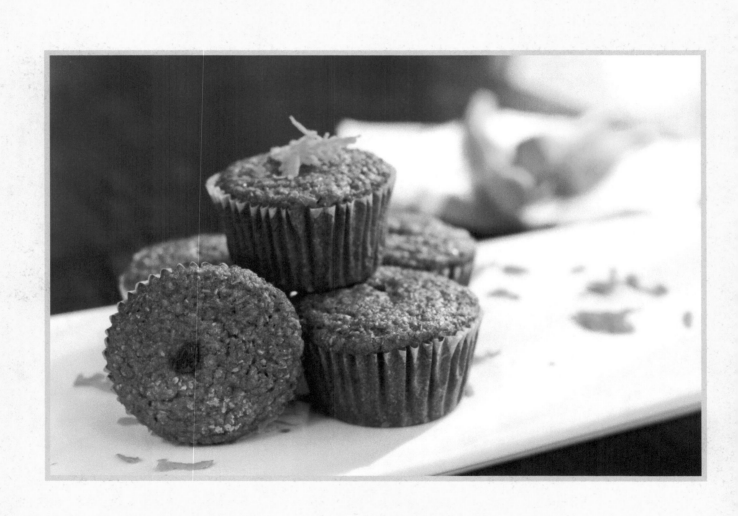

Healthy Goodies

Here are some guilt-free desserts which are favorites of my clients and family. They represent imaginative baking and are made up of quality, available ingredients. I believe they will become favorites of yours too.

The Special Occasion Carrot Cake always makes my family smile when I serve it. My daughter, niece and daughter-in-law each have requested I make the cake for their special gatherings and I have done so with much love. My second grandson, Luca Hudson, just turned one year of age and I baked this in the shape of a "1" for his party. It's more labor than most cakes, but WOW to the outcome. Prepping the carrots the day before can lessen that time.

With less processed sugar, organic eggs and 4 cups of shredded carrots and unsweetened coconut, it's extremely moist and almost tropical. It's mouth watering delicious and does not even need the frosting. (But go for it anyway.)

Biscotti are hand-crafted and very creative to make. You must make them with passion and care to really get an excellent finished product. There are many different combinations of ingredients in Biscotti to choose from, and some are not even on the sweet side.

My fruit and nut biscotti are wholesome and satisfying. I adore having one with tea with a girlfriend for a mid-day stress reliever. My husband loves them with breakfast. We made them everyday in our store and the plate was always empty. The cacao sweet nibs are an important superfood and they are a new addition to this 1998 recipe. These cookies can be easily converted to gluten-free, and no nuts.

Rustic Chocolate-Prune Nut Bars or cake with walnuts reminds us of a European version minus the white flour/white sugar. Prunes are so rich in vitamins and minerals, and paired with a flour of substance, unprocessed sugar, organic chocolate, and mineral rich walnuts, this dessert packs power. You're going to be pleasantly surprised here.

While traveling years ago, I found an old copy in an antique store of *The Ladies Home Journal* from June 1922. The header stood out; For a healthier today and tomorrow. The advertisement for *Sunset Prunes* reads, "The wealth of the nation tomorrow hinges on the health of the children today. Good health is the youth birth-right of every child. Do mothers realize how important prunes are? Prunes are rich in fruit sugar, which means energy. They are rich in tonic iron. That means greater strength- resistance to disease. And too, these natural, juicy sweet meats provide a laxative made in nature's own pharmacy." How appropriate was that **91 years** ago?

I like to end here with one of my favorite passages from a treasured book *Nourishing Wisdom* by Marc David. The chapter entitled "The Elements of Sweetness" reads;

> "In the spiritual tradition of India, it is said that if you could taste the soul, it would be sweet. Indeed, the human condition in some of its most precious moments is perceived as "sweet": "the sweet life", our "sweetheart", "sweet dreams", or "the sweet smell of success". Sweetness is an experience and food is just the doorway that leads us there. Food happens to be the most available form of the sweet experience. Sugary food is one of the most popular forms of substitute love. Its effect is even more potent when combined with the love-inducing chemicals in chocolate. This yearning for sweetness is simply the heart's desire to smile."

So bake with crazy love, and smile.

Special Occasion Carrot Cake

Yield: 2, 9-inch round cakes, 12-14 servings

Ingredients:

4 cups organic carrots (about 6 carrots), peeled and grated

1¼ cups whole wheat pastry flour

1¼ cups unbleached white flour

¼ cup unsweetened shredded coconut

2 teaspoons baking soda

2 teaspoons baking powder

4 large organic eggs, room temperature

1½ cups organic light brown sugar

1 teaspoon pure vanilla extract

1 cup safflower oil or melted organic unsalted butter

¼ cup fresh or canned pineapple, pureed or mashed

1 cup *Apple-Apricot Sauce* by *Santa-Cruz Organic*

1 cup walnuts, small chop

Spices:

1 teaspoon ground cinnamon

¼ teaspoon ground cardamom

¼ teaspoon ground ginger

⅛ teaspoon ground nutmeg

⅛ teaspoon ground mace

For the pans:

1 tablespoon of natural buttery spread, like *Earth Balance*

2 tablespoons white flour for dusting

20-inch piece of natural parchment paper, cut in half

Procedure:

1. Preheat oven to 350 degrees.
2. To prepare your pans, cut parchment paper to fit the inside circumference of each pan. Lightly grease the bottom of each cake pan and the bottom of paper liner with a natural buttery spread. Dust with the 2 tablespoons of white flour. Shake off excess and set aside.
3. Grate the carrots on a hand grater (using large holes) or shred using the blade for the food processor. Set aside.
4. In a large mixing bowl, stir to incorporate first 6 ingredients.
5. In a medium bowl and with an electric mixture (or by hand), beat eggs and sugar until fluffy, about 1 minute. Add vanilla and stir in oil or butter and blend well. Mix in pineapple.
6. Stir the remaining ingredients into the dry mixture to incorporate well being cautious not to over mix. Fold in carrots, applesauce, and walnuts.
7. Pour into the prepared pans and bake for 40-45 minutes, until done. It will have a medium golden color. Use a toothpick to insert towards the middle to test for doneness. I use the bounce back test with my finger.

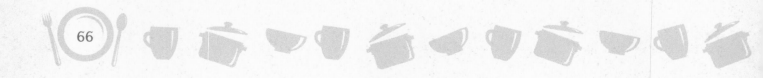

Orange Cream Cheese Frosting

Yield: 2 cups

Ingredients

2, 8-ounce packages organic cream cheese (can be light cream cheese), room temperature
1 stick organic unsalted butter, room temperature
1 teaspoon vanilla extract
1 organic orange, zested and juiced to yield ¼-½ cup fresh juice
1 pound Confectioner's sugar
1 teaspoon vanilla extract

Optional
2 cups chopped pecans for around the edges of cake

Procedure

1. Cream together softened cream cheese and butter. Add vanilla and orange zest.
2. Slowly add in sugar, ½ cup at a time, alternating it with the orange juice.
3. Blend until smooth. Add more juice if needed to produce a creamy texture.
4. Assemble cake and frost up the sides. Decorate with the chopped pecans.

Cook's Notes:

- Using organic ingredients makes for a more delicious taste and a guiltless experience.
- Both the cake and the frosting freeze well. Freeze each separately and frost when ready to serve.
- When I am not making this cake for a special occasion, I bake it in 2, 8-inch spring-form cake pans. I freeze one, and then I have one great dessert for an unplanned casual occasion. It's a special treat however you plan it.
- There are many coconut products on the market today. My choice is *Woodstock Organic Shredded Coconut*. It tastes delicious and they support the *American Farmland Trust*.

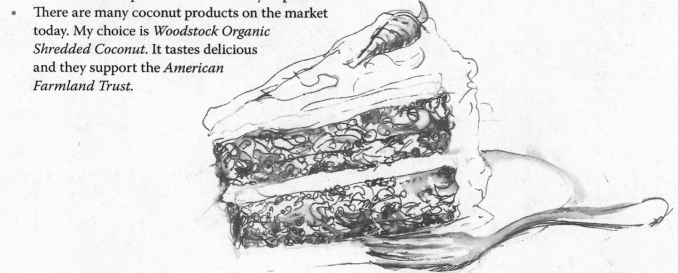

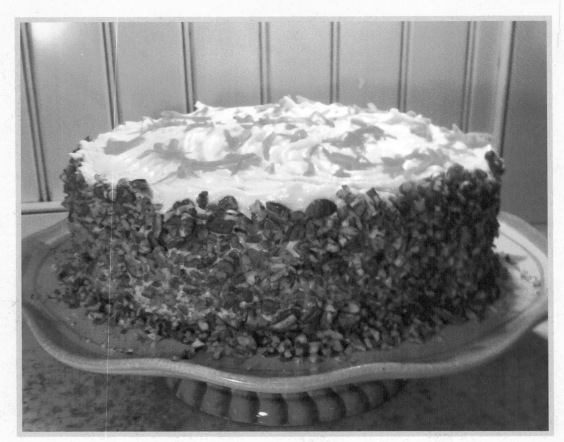

Special Occasion Carrot Cake

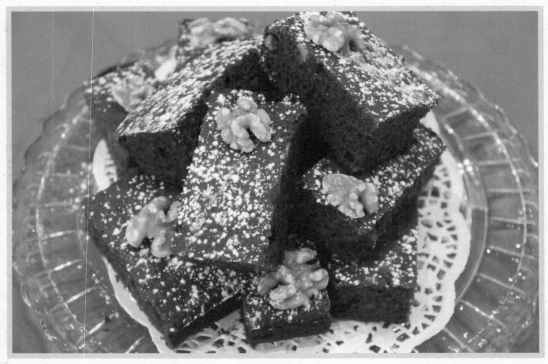

Rustic Chocolate-Prune Nut Bars

Rustic Chocolate-Prune Nut Bars

Yield: 16 bars or 1, 9 –inch round cake

Ingredients:

1 cup prune puree (from about 22 pitted prunes)
2 square (2 ounces) unsweetened dark chocolate
1½ cups whole wheat or spelt flour
1 teaspoon baking powder
½ teaspoon baking soda
¼ cup unsweetened Dutch-processed cocoa, sifted
¼ teaspoon sea salt
1 teaspoon ground cinnamon
¼ teaspoon ground cardamom
¼ teaspoon ground mace

6 tablespoons organic unsalted butter, softened to room temperature
1 cup natural sugar
2 large eggs, room temperature
1 teaspoon pure vanilla extract
½ cup whole milk or unsweetened almond milk
1 cup walnuts, small chop

Optional garnish:
Powdered confectioner's sugar for a dusting on top
1 cup raspberries for plate decoration

Procedure:

1. Preheat oven to 350 degrees.
2. To prepare your pan, cut parchment paper to fit the inside of a 9- x- 13- inch shallow rectangular pan. Lightly grease the bottom of pan and the bottom of paper liner with a natural buttery spread. Set the pan aside.
3. Rinse and drain prunes. In a 4-quart saucepan, bring 3½ cups of water to a rapid boil. Add prunes and lower to simmer for 20 minutes, or until tender. Drain the prunes over a bowl - preferably a bowl with a pouring spout. Save all of the juice after straining. Cool a few minutes before pureeing.
4. In a food processor puree the prunes with half of the prune juice until creamy. Keep adding juice slowly, just until you reach this consistency. It should have no lumps and look like melted chocolate. Scrape out 1 cup for the cake recipe. You can save the rest of prune puree for a yummy treat at breakfast or just about any time.
5. Place the chocolate in a small saucepan, a double boiler, or place in a covered bowl in the microwave. Melt the chocolate (it should take about 2 minutes) and then set aside to cool. You will need a small spatula to scrape out.
6. In a medium sized mixing bowl, mix the flour, baking soda, baking powder, spices and sifted cocoa - which you can sift right over this bowl.
7. In a slightly larger bowl with an electric hand mixer (or by hand), cream butter and sugar until fluffy. Beat in eggs, one at a time. Add the vanilla and the cooled, melted chocolate.
8. On low speed, add half the flour alternatively with the milk, starting and ending with flour.
9. Stir in prune puree and nuts. Turn batter into prepared pan and smooth the top.
10. Bake for 30-35 minutes or until top bounces back when lightly pressed with fingertip.

Cook's Notes:

- If making into a cake, follow #2 under procedure, using a- 9-inch round cake pan. Baking time will be the same
- I suggest fair trade cocoa by *Equal Exchange* or *Rapunzel*.
- Purchase prunes without sulfates or other chemical additives. Organic tastes best
- Extra prune puree will last up to 4 weeks in refrigerator.

This recipe was adapted from *Maida Heatter's Book of Great Chocolate Desserts*

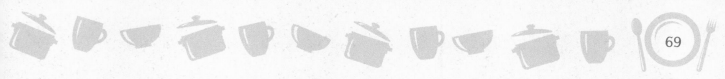

Treasured Biscotti

Biscotti are the official Italian "dunking cookies." The biscotti cookie has been around for centuries. They were originally made as a long-shelf life food for Roman soldiers, sailors and travelers. They become crisper when twice baked, removing all moisture and becoming a cracker-like food. They can stay fresh for 2 months without preservatives or additives. (But do store in a tight sealed container).

Biscotti traces its origins to Roman times. After the fall of the Roman Empire, the biscotti became a staple in Tuscan cities and spread throughout the Italian peninsula. Biscotti became so popular that every province developed their own flavored version. It was the favorite of Christopher Columbus, who brought the long lasting biscotti to the new world.

In my culinary career, I set out to create guilt-free biscotti for my own customers. I wanted to incorporate the goodness of nuts and fruits. I used dried fruits for an extended shelf life and preferred a more wholesome flour than the white variety. I wanted them to be crispy and rustic and hit the spot when you wanted a healthier treat. I did accomplish this and this recipe became a success for the store.

It's a treasured gift to give to those I love during holiday time. This recipe of biscotti arranges perfectly into antique tins. During the year I do take time to shop for and collect special colorful designed tins, looking for them in antique stores, second hand stores, consignment stores, craft fairs and garage sales.

During summer months, I love to bake lemon blueberry cornmeal biscotti with a lemon glaze. Biscotti also make a great school snack for kids when using wholesome flours, low sugar and a protein like almond or sunflower butter. At home use peanut butter for kids in the mix (most schools now will not allow that ingredient), it makes yummy biscotti for them.

Hopefully my healthy version will be a favorite of yours. Bake them with a warm and generous heart and enjoy this gratifying Italian treat.

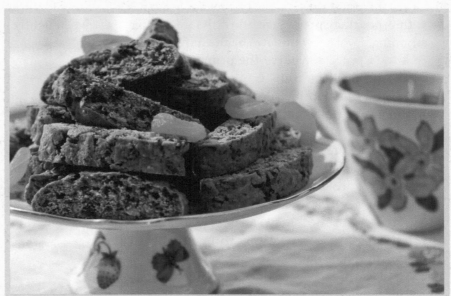

Fruit and Nut Biscotti with Raw Cacao Nibs

Yield: 22 large or 45 medium biscotti

Dry Ingredients:

½ cup almonds, roasted and chopped
¼ cup almond meal
1 cup spelt flour
1 cup barley flour
1 teaspoon baking powder
1 teaspoon baking soda
½ teaspoon sea salt
1 teaspoon ground cinnamon
½ teaspoon ground cardamom
½ cup natural sugar

Wet ingredients:

1 large egg plus 2 egg whites
3 tablespoons safflower oil
¼ cup grade B maple syrup
1½ teaspoons almond extract
1½ teaspoons pure vanilla extract
½ cup unsulfured apricots, thinly sliced into small slivers
½ cup currants
1 cup organic raw cacao nibs

Procedure:

1. Preheat oven to 350 degrees. Cut parchment paper to fit sheet pan. Lightly oil.
2. Roast almonds in the oven for 8 minutes or on stovetop for 6 minutes, shaking the pan while roasting for even cooking. Cool for 10 minutes. Hand-chop into thin slivers.
3. In a large mixing bowl combine all dry ingredients.
4. In a separate small bowl beat eggs together.
5. Whisk oil and maple syrup to emulsify. Add the vanilla and the egg mixture. Beat 2 minutes or until well blended.
6. Mix the wet ingredients into the dry with a large spatula or wooden spoon until just combined. It will feel dry. Fold in the apricots, currants and cacao nibs.
7. On prepared baking sheet with oiled hands, form and shape dough into 2 slightly flattened logs. By eye, measure each log 14 x 2½ inches for the large biscotti or 12 x 2 inches for the medium. Leave 3-4 inches between logs for expansion and 2 inches on each top and bottom of pan.
8. Bake 25 minutes or until slightly firm to your touch. Cool 30 minutes on sheet pan or overnight before slicing.
9. Preheat (or reduce) oven to 325 degrees.
10. Using a cutting board, cut biscotti diagonally into ½-inch pieces.
11. Arrange biscotti cut-side down. Bake for 5 minutes on each side until crisp. Cool again before handling or packaging.

Cook's Notes:

- Almond meal is now available in healthy marketplaces. You can make it yourself by using a small food processor or other chopping machine. Simply chop until you see the consistence of grainy flour.
- You can use a combination of other flours here but you want a rustic product so stay with the whole grains.
- Some suggestions for natural dry sugar are: dark or light coconut sugar, organic coconut palm sugar, date sugar, sucanut, organic granulated sugar, and organic brown sugar.
- You can substitute the cacao nibs with 1 cup semi-sweet chocolate chips or carob chips. However the nibs are high in antioxidants and magnesium.
- You can order quality apricots online at *Vitacost.com* and certified organic raw cacao nibs at *Amazon.com*.

Well Stocked Healthy Pantry

For me, all roads lead to a well-stocked pantry. With today's busy schedule, being organized just makes sense, plus, it will save you time in the long run. As you have read in this book, healthy eating is about cooking fresh and staying close to Mother Nature. Most of the pantry items listed below are dried and I've placed them in a group called "The Foods of Importance." Beans, legumes, whole grains, nuts, seeds, herbs, spices, and sea vegetables are all known for longevity. For these items, bulk buying makes sense both economically and ecologically.

Visualize and plan your meals

Make a plan to sit down with your family during the weekend to figure out how many meals you'll need to prepare for the week ahead. I tell the students and parents I work with, "you must have a plan first."

When organizing your meals, think seasonally! You'll discover better quality and fresher ingredients. Keep in mind that the rotation of foods is important to the nutrition of the body. You'll discover better quality and fresher ingredients. Plus, trying different groups of foods keeps meals exciting.

Try choosing from the "Rainbow Diet," matching color to important food groups. For example, plan your menu to include green, yellow, perhaps some purple from cabbage, and orange from sweet potato. Then, match the vegetables up with a protein. Our needs change as our life experiences change. Remember that diet is an ongoing discovery and rotating what you consume will help you reap all the nutritional benefits.

For well-balanced meals, I like to choose a recipe that is versatile and can be used for breakfast, lunch, and dinner. Veggie burgers or a frittata, three-bean chili with quinoa and crisp corn chips on the side are always nice choices. Because of our easy access to the Internet, we are blessed to have so many recipes at our fingertips. If you shop on the weekends, try to plan dishes that require a variety of fresh ingredients for the early parts of the week and choose meals that rely primarily on more dried goods for later in the week. Vegetarian dishes are a wonderful choice because they tend to last a bit longer than meat and fish dishes, which tend to be more perishable.

Useful tips on leftovers

Make a double batch of rice or beans when making your meals so they can be used for soups and salads later in the week. I like serving leftovers with a fresh, raw salad or vegetable to spark up the meal and nutritional value. Some sprouts and garnishes are excellent choices here.

Bring everyone around the table to get involve in the planning

Working with multiple families through the years, I've noticed when children are involved in making the menu and participate in the cutting of veggies or using the salad spinner, they tend to eat the meals they helped to prepare. There is power in this type of group planning.

The Happy Pantry

This is a long cabinet in my kitchen that I converted into a pantry for my favorite healthy items. It sits directly on the counter. I also have additional storage in a closet close by. Consider yourself fortunate if you have a nice size pantry right in the kitchen! You may have shelves in your basement for addition items. There are many stores today that carry stainless steel racks, slender china cabinets, cabinets with glass fronts, etc. They are all very useful. The point is, you can find a special place to keep all these products available at a moments notice.

Spice Medicine

The resurgence of herbal medicine, also called "Spice Medicine," combined with the environmental movement and the holistic principle of "natural is better," has brought herbs and spices to the fore-front once again.

In our modern kitchen we can capture the thrill of the spice trade with quality spices in a variety of colors and textures. Cooking with herbs has taken on a new importance with our awareness of reducing salt and fat in the diet. Herbs can be used to enliven flavors in many dishes with aroma, flavor, and color when salt and fat are reduced in the recipe. In addition, the spice may increase the body's ability to digest fat. The gathering of herbs and spices is a delightful, soulful experience that stimulates the senses. Spice stories were woven more intimately into the fabric of daily life in ancient times.

Spice and Herb Facts

- The difference between an herb and a spice is that an herb is an aromatic leaf, like fresh parsley, and a spice stems from a pungent seed, root, or bark, such as cinnamon.
- Most herbs stimulate the senses and act as food for the body. They maintain wellness in the prevention of disease and are rich in antioxidants, helping to neutralize free radicals.
- All spices are not created equal. Purchase organic when possible and choose smaller jars over large containers – especially those sold in large chain stores. Since spices can go rancid and collect mold, you won't want to keep them more than one year.
- Remember to date your spices with a small sticker on the back or top of the jar. This will help reduce any confusion about when you may have purchased them.

These are my personal choices for your pantry. Take time to build your personal inventory. Have fun and get creative while boosting your nutrition with the following ingredients:

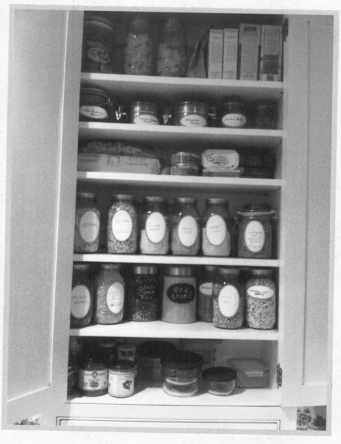

Healthier Salts

Atlantic Sea Salt
Bragg's Sprinkle 24 Herbs and Spices
Celtic Sea Salt
Himalayan Sea Salt
Herbamare

Spices

Anise
Basil
Black Pepper
Caraway seeds
Cayenne pepper
Chili Powder
Chipotle pepper
Coriander
Curry
Dill
Fennel seeds
Ground Fennel
Mustard Seeds
Oregano
Paprika
Thyme
Turmeric

Baking Spices

Allspice
Cardamom
Cinnamon
Cloves
Ginger
Nutmeg

Fair Trade Cocoa

Cacao Nibs

Sweeteners

Barley Malt
Brown Rice Syrup
Coconut Sugar
Date Sugar
Maple Sugar
Maple Syrup
Molasses
Rapadura
Raw Honey
Sucanut
Wild Flower Local Honey

Condiments/ Dry Goods

Almonds
Applesauce
Bran Cereal
Brazil Nuts
Canned Tuna (White Albacore)
Chia Seeds
Cranberries
Dark Chocolate
Dijon Mustard
Ghee
Strained Tomatoes
Green/Black Olives
Organic Almond Butter
Capers
Organic Peanut Butter
Prunes
Raisins
Sesame seeds
Sesame Tahini
Stone Ground Mustard
Walnuts

Baking Flours

Almond Flour
Amaranth Flour
Arrowroot
Barley Flour
Brown Rice Flour
Buckwheat Flour
Coconut Flour
Cornmeal
Garbanzo Bean Flour
Spelt Flour
Whole Wheat Pastry Flour

Dairy Alternatives

Almond/Rice Milk
Coconut Milk
Hemp/Oat Milk

Oils/Vinegars

Apple Cider Vinegar
Balsamic Vinegar
Brown Rice Vinegar
Organic Cold-Pressed Olive Oil
Grape Seed Oil
Safflower Oil
Organic Coconut Oil
Pure Sesame Oil
White Champagne vinegar

Refrigerator Staples

Bragg's Liquid Amino Acids
Ground Flax Seeds
Maine Coast Sea Seasoning; Kelp and Dulse
    seaweed shakers
Miso - Sweet White
Organic Cage-free Eggs
Organic Milk
Tamari – Reduced Sodium
Organic, Unsalted Butter
Prepared Horseradish
Sauerkraut
Vegenaise

Freezer Staples

Buckwheat Multigrain Waffles
Edamame
Frozen Fruit
Organic Corn
Organic Peas
Wild Blueberries

This is my Healthy Well-Stocked Healthy Pantry List

Start with a few items from each category and work towards purchasing all.

The Japanese and Chinese Pantry

The Well-Stocked Japanese Pantry

Bamboo Rolling Mat - A tightly woven mat used for rolling sushi or California rolls.

Brown Rice Vinegar - Sweeter than cider vinegar. Use in salad and rice dishes.

Mirin – A sweet cooking wine made from glutinous rice. Best used for cooking purposes.

Nori - Paper-thin sheets of seaweed used as the edible wrapper in sushi or California rolls.

Organic Brown Rice - Short and long-grain, a staple food for fried rice or beans.

Organic Sesame Oil - Extremely healthy oil derived from tiny white sesame seeds.

Organic Tamari - Gluten-free soy sauce, naturally brewed from whole soybeans.

Sesame seeds - Mild nut-like flavor, intensified when toasted.

Shoyu - Light and flavorful Japanese soy sauce.

Soba Noodles - Multiple varieties made from any one of the following combinations: 100% buckwheat, a blend of wheat and buckwheat flours, or a combination including wild yam or lotus root. Use in hot and cold dishes.

Toasted Sesame Oil - Dark, rich flavor. Use as a seasoning oil just before serving.

Udon - Long, round noodles similar to spaghetti. Mild in taste, blends well with all dishes.

Umeboshi - Salt-cured plums known to aid digestion.

Ume Plum Vinegar - A tart, salty vinegar made from Ume plums.

Wasabi - Potent Japanese green horseradish, traditionally served with sushi.

Freezer Item

Edamame - Green soybeans, purchase in the pod or shelled.

Refrigerated Perishables

Daikon Root - A large, white Japanese radish with a sweet, pungent taste and a crisp texture.

Garlic - Fresh only. Mince and stir into sauté or blend into dressings.

Ginger - Fresh only. Choose firm, shiny skin. Grate or chop to use in all Asian cooking.

Miso - Fermented paste made from a mixture of soybeans and grain. Varieties include Sweet White and Hearty Red. Use in sauces.

Scallions – Also called green onions, use as garnish or in stir-fries.

Wonton and Spring Roll Wrappers - Sold fresh in packages. Use to wrap fillings for spring rolls and dumplings. They become crispy when baked.

The Well-Stocked Chinese Pantry

Agar-Agar - A clear thickening agent made from seaweed.

Arrowroot - A natural thickener. Use in sauces.

Cellophane Noodles - Clear, dried noodles. Use in spring rolls. Boil or soak in hot water to soften.

Cilantro - Often called "Chinese parsley." Has a distinct flavor and is packed with medicinal properties.

Coconut Milk - Made from fresh coconut meat. Has a creamy, rich texture.

Coriander - The dried seed of the cilantro plant. Use in sautés or stir-fries.

Five-Spice Powder - A blend of warm, aromatic spices. Use sparingly in savory dishes.

Hoisin Sauce - A thick sauce that is sweet with a slightly spicy, garlicky flavor. Use sparingly.

Mung Bean Pasta – Delicate wheat-free pasta made from mung beans. Enjoy with stir-fries.

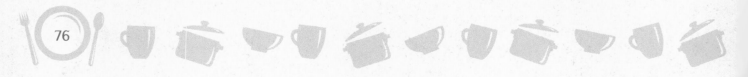

Bok Choy – A sweet-tasting cruciferous vegetable that comes in two sizes, baby and regular. Eat raw or cooked.

Lemongrass - Sold in stalks. Has a sharp, citrus flavor and fragrance. Use inner bulb.

Napa Cabbage - Pale green, delicately flavored; the most popular vegetable in China.

Essential Items for the Stir-Fry

The wok is the main cooking vessel for the stir-fry. An authentic wok is made from black carbon steel and needs special care. Some fun cooking utensils you may want to purchase for this style of cooking include: a wooden rice paddle/spoon, a wedge shaped metal scoop, and spring-loaded tongs.

Since natural cooking methods don't rely on the deep-frying methods that are authentic in Asian cooking, I use a large skillet pan rather than a wok. A few tablespoons of pure sesame oil in the beginning of the sauté, plus one or two at the end to toss the noodles, is all that is needed. Whatever instrument you choose to use, enjoy the experience, it's fun and so creative!

Follow Me to the Bean Buzz:
Amazing Health Benefits and Facts

Research has indicated that foods such as legumes provide more than sustenance, some may actually help prevent chronic diseases. They are one of the most versatile, nourishing, and least expensive foods that exist. They have a high-protein content and are a good source of iron and key nutrients. Containing zero cholesterol and no saturated fat, they are among the highest sources of antioxidants. Legumes are a tonic food for your kidneys and can also help with stabilizing blood sugar levels. When paired with a grain, they are considered a whole-food, for example: black beans and rice or hummus on a whole-wheat pita.

Rebecca Wood, the author of many award-winning books, is an authority on beans and grains. She teaches that beans support your endurance and build energy. She sees the wonder of beans as a "universal image of nurture."

> For millennia, farmers have dried legumes in the field and then shelled, cleaned, and stored them. It's the same today. Beans are unrefined, and they're not washed, parched, polished, gassed, preserved, or colored. Providing they're organic and not genetically modified, their earthly sweetness is utterly unadulterated. No wonder they are so satisfying.[1]

Beans, lentils, and peas all fall under the term legumes, but they grow and look differently. Beans and peas are the edible seeds of *leguminous plants*, a large grow of flowering plants that produce double-stemmed pods with a single row of seeds. Belonging to this group are garden peas, snow peas, snap peas, chickpeas, and fava beans. The mung bean, soybean, adzuki bean, black-eyed pea, and runner beans are many varieties of "boutique" beans.

Commonly recognized peas are the green and yellow split pea. Lentils such as brown, green, red, and yellow have a long history in the world. The lentil is thought to be the oldest legume, having been cultivated starting as far back as c. 7000 BC. Legumes, as well as herbs and spices, were an old form of currency.

If you haven't tasted a chickpea (also called garbanzo) cooked from scratch, you are depriving yourself of a delicious and nutritious treat. Once you go the extra mile, there's no going back to the can. Canned beans often trap gas inside the container without oxygen. There may be times of necessity where it will be less stressful to reach for the canned version. The brand *Eden* uses cans with a BPA-free coating. Plus, their beans are cooked with a piece of Kombu seaweed in which I explain the benefits below. You can also find beans sold in paper cartons by different companies.

What I love about the study of beans is that every culture around the world has its own authentic bean to boast about, and their stories are rich in history. While visiting New Orleans for the first time, *Red Beans and Rice* was a must to try. I certainty savored the spices of their culture. It was a memorable dish, yet so simple. Today the global market offers great diversity among legumes. For me, it's endlessly fascinating to choose from a vast variety of different shapes, sizes, and colors to create many delicious ethnic dishes from around the world.

---

[1] http://www.rwood.com/Articles/Beans_Build_Energy.htm

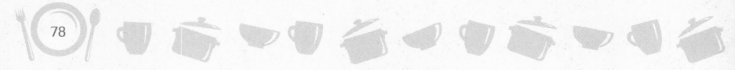

Encouraging Tips from the Chef

Beans can be divided into those that need no soaking and those that do. All beans need washing. Although soaking is not essential for every type of legume, they can all benefit from it. Soaking shortens the cooking time and improves digestibility. Going one step further, sprouting beans increases their digestibility even more and shortens cooking time as well.

To soak or not to soak

1. Soaking breaks down the indigestible sugars that may cause gas.
2. Soaking softens beans and makes them easier to cook.
3. While soaking, beans absorb enough moisture to then double in volume and weight.
4. For anyone in the family with compromised health, soaking promotes greater digestibility.
5. Personally I get motivated to cook beans when I see them soaking in a beautiful bowl.

How to soak

1. Pick over the beans thoroughly. I like to put the darker beans on white wax paper or a light flat platter to clearly see if they have pebbles, small stones, or clumps of dirt.
2. Put them in a strainer and place the strainer in tepid water in a large bowl and swish around. Some tiny bits may float to the top. These may be older beans or beans that were harvested prematurely. Simply discard them. I suggest buying another brand if this happens often. For that reason, purchase beans from a bulk bin or in a see-through wrapper.
3. The traditional "long soak method" or "cold method" is to soak the beans overnight. Pour enough water to cover 3-4 inches over the top of the washed beans. Let sit uncovered for 6-8 hours. If for some reason your plans change and you cannot get to cooking the beans, simply change the water once a day (this will prevent fermentation) until you're ready to cook.
4. For the "short soaking method" or "hot method," place the picked over and washed beans in a 4-quart saucepan and add hot water to cover 2-3 inches and bring slowly to a boil. Boil for 5 minutes and turn off the flame. Let the beans soak in the hot water, covered, for 2 hours. After soaking, drain and discard the soaking water and rinse beans in tepid water. Do not cook beans in the water used to soak them. Proceed with your recipe instructions.

Beans that need no soaking

Times listed below are approximate cooking times. Please take into consideration your stove temperature and whether or not you use gas or electric. Legumes should be firm and tender but not mushy. After bringing beans to a boil, reduce heat and simmer for individual times stated below.

Adzuki beans - 1 hour
Green lentils - 30-45 minutes
Red lentils - 20 minutes
Split peas (yellow/green) - 1¼-1½ hours

Beans that need soaking

After bringing beans to a boil, reduce heat to a slow boil for individual times stated below.

Black Beans - 50-60 minutes
Black-eyed peas - 35 minutes

Chickpeas - 1½-2 hours
Kidney - 50-60 minutes
Lima (large and small) - 60-70 minutes
Navy - 45 minutes
Pinto - 50 minutes

Please note to always stir beans while cooking. Cooking times may vary according to the age of the bean. Since beans become tougher as they age, the older they are, the longer they need to cook. Test 20 minutes before suggested finishing time above. Keep in mind that 1 cup of dried beans yields 2 ½-3 cups cooked. It's a good idea to cook more than you will need for one meal, however, it is easy to go overboard and cook more than you will be able to use.

My Secret Ingredient in Cooking Beans

There is a premium quality dried seaweed called "Kombu" that I use in the bean and legume cooking water. Kombu is an edible ocean plant that is sold in health food stores and many natural markets such as *Whole Foods* and major markets like *Fairway*. Asian markets sell dried Kombu, but I suggest buying a brand like *Emerald Cove*, which has no GMO'S. Look for a package that weighs about 2 ounces. If you're using it every week, the package will last approximately 5-6 months.

To start, cut or tear a tiny piece the size of your pinky finger. Rinse it well and place in the cooking water with your beans or legumes. Allow it to remain during the entire time the legumes cook. When the soup is finished, puree half the soup with the Kombu. If you're not pureeing the soup, just break up the softened piece with a fork, or cut with a knife, and use in the soup. It will look like the herb parsley in the soup. Kombu has a pleasant, almost sweet, taste. The small piece of seaweed that you started with is a potent, mineral-rich sea vegetable that will remove the gas from the beans while they're cooking. One of its greatest properties is that it pulls toxins from the body, which is extremely helpful to a person who has finished chemotherapy.

Cooking the Beans
For Stove-Top Cooking:

- Start the beans cooking in tepid water (not cold), or low-sodium stock. The use of aromatic vegetables such as, onions, carrots, celery, and herbs like thyme and bay leaves, will add additional flavor.
- The water will start to foam in the beginning. The foam is the protein in the beans. Simply skim off just once or twice.
- Tilt the lid of the pot slightly to prevent boiling over.
- Beans should start with a rolling boil for 20 minutes, then lower temperature to a medium boil for another 20 minutes, finally ending with a simmer for the remainder of time.
- If water level goes down, add boiling water as needed.
- Stir occasionally for even cooking.
- Never add salt or anything acidic while the beans cook such as tomatoes, vinegar, wine, molasses, or citrus juices. Add salt after the beans are almost tender.
- To test for doneness try a few beans from different areas in the pot, since some may be tender and some not. If they are not proper consistency, continue to cook.
- When cooling, keep the beans in the cooking liquid to prevent them from drying out as well as preventing the skins from splitting or bursting.
- If you're reheating beans, add a tablespoon or two of water or reserved cooking liquid. As beans cool, they will absorb any leftover liquid that may still be there.

Pressure Cookers

Using a pressure cooker is a time-efficient cooking method. The pressure cooker turns out a lentil soup in 7 minutes and a steamed bread pudding in well under an hour. This is because it cooks food at higher-than-standard boiling-point temperature.

Once the lid is locked into place, the cooker is set over high heat and boiling liquid produces steam. Since the steam is sealed inside, pressure builds and internal temperature rises, increasing the boiling point. Under high pressure, the fiber in the food is softened and flavors mingle in record time. I personally do not use a pressure cooker. I may be old fashioned but the stovetop works well for me. I love the process of stirring the beans and smelling them as they cook. For the most inspiring information on the pressure cooker, take a look at the highly acclaimed book *Cooking under Pressure,* by award-winning cookbook author Lorna J. Sass, Ph.D.

How to Store Beans
Dried Beans

- I prefer to store beans and legumes in tight airtight glass containers. In my *Well-Stocked Healthy Pantry List* in this book, you'll find a picture of the jars I store in. They are mason jars and various glass jars I washed out from pickles, sauces, etc.
- Contents of packages bought several months apart should not be mixed when storing, since older beans will take longer to cook.
- Move your beans around to inspire you to cook certain ethnic dishes.
- Out of site means out of mind, so keep a few jars right on the counter every week.

Cooked Beans

- Should you cook more beans than you need for a given recipe, they'll keep in the refrigerator for up to three days. They can also be frozen up to three months. Simply divide your cooked beans in portion sizes or recipe-size containers.
- Bean soups will keep in the freezer for three months.

Smart Bean Tips

- Some stores sell eye-catching mixes of different beans. Since beans require different soaking and cooking times, mixing them together targets the uninformed cook, so they are not always a wise choice.
- If you're transitioning your diet to a more wholesome one, and you're just learning about and trying new beans, consume in small amounts at first, ½ cup or less.
- When beans are a regular part of the diet, our systems adapt to them and digestion becomes easier.
- Keep your meals simple. When you first have legumes, omit potatoes, fruit, sweeteners, (such as molasses with baked beans), or desserts in the same meal.
- Add salt or tamari near the end of cooking.
- Use the spices turmeric, cumin, coriander, ginger, and garlic as standard spices when cooking beans to help aid in digestibility.
- Miso, sauerkraut, and yogurt are good to serve in the same meal with beans because they are foods that aid in digestion.
- Drinking with meals inhibits digestion to some extent. When we drink with our meals, the time that the food spends in our mouth is much shorter. Less saliva is produced and the food is less thoroughly chewed. Digestive enzymes in the mouth, stomach, and intestines are diluted and thus, digestion is delayed. Also, the stomach must make more acid to retain the proper environment for digestion. All of these factors

increase the likelihood of fermentation and gas on the digestive system. So, when starting to include all of the above in your diet, take this great advice from many top health practitioners. In other cultures this is a way of life.

Yummy Suggestions For These Robust Friends

- Legumes and beans can be pureed into a spread for appetizers and sandwiches.
- Mash and use to fill tortillas for breakfast, lunch, or dinner.
- Cook, puree and add to thicken soups.
- Add to stews for extra protein and richness.
- Bean and lentil salads are versatile and delicious for every season.
- What would a classic Chili dish be without hearty, flavorful beans

Get on the Bean Wagon - the benefits are endless and the tastes are divine!!

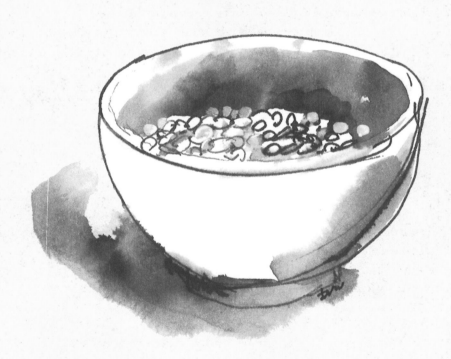

Say No to GMO

Genetic Engineering (GE) is an experimental technology that involves the artificial transfer of genetic material, or DNA, between unrelated species. GE can combine species that would never combine naturally. For the sake of short-term profits, the biotech industry is engineering plants with genes from *bacteria, viruses, insects, animals and even humans,* into the DNA of a food crop or animal to introduce a new trait. There are many potential health risks associated with GE food such as infertility, immune problems, accelerated aging, faulty insulin regulation, and changes in major organ systems and the gastrointestinal tract.

Unfortunately, food companies who make products that contain genetically modified organisms (GMO's) are not required to include that on the label. To avoid any genetically modified (GM) ingredients it is suggested to buy products that are labeled "100% organic", or look for the Non-GMO Project Verified Seal. You should avoid items that are made with ingredients from the eight GM food crops which are Corn, Soybeans, Canola, Cottonseed, Sugar Beets, most Hawaiian Papaya and some Zucchini and Yellow Squash. If a non-organic product made in North America lists "sugar" as an ingredient (not pure cane sugar), then it is most likely a combination of sugar from both sugar cane and GM sugar beets. When buying dairy products, look for labels stating No *rBGH, rBST,* or artificial hormones, otherwise those products may have been made from cows that were injected with GM bovine growth hormone. If you are buying any processed food, it is highly likely that you are eating GE foods every day. You can get involved on many levels to help spread the word!

The following is a list of invisible GM ingredients, which are often hidden in processed foods:

Aspartame	cysteine	hydrogenated starch	milo starch	soy sauce
baking powder	dextrin	hydrolyzed	modified food starch	starch
canola oil	dextrose	vegetable protein	modified starch	stearic acid
caramel color	diacetyl	inositol	mono and	sugar (unless cane)
cellulose	diglyceride	inverse syrup	triglyceride	tamari
citric acid	Equal	inversol	monosodium	tempeh
cobalamin	erythritol	invert sugar	glutamate (MSG)	teriyaki marinade
(Vit. B12)	food starch	isoflavones	Nutrasweet	textured vegetable
colorose	fructose (any form)	lactic acid	oleic acid	protein
condensed milk	glucose	lecithin	phenylalanine	threonine
confectioner's	glutamate	leucine	phytic acid	tocopherols (vit E)
sugar	glutamic acid	lysine	protein isolate	tofu
corn flour	gluten	malt	shoyu	trehalose
corn masa	glycerides	malt extract	sorbitol	triglyceride
corn meal	glycerin	malt syrup	soy flour	vegetable fat
corn oil	glycerol	maltitol	soy isolates	vegetable oil
corn sugar	glycerol monooleate	maltodextrin	soy lecithin	vitamin B12
corn syrup	glycine	maltose	soy milk	vitamin E
cornstarch	hemicellulose	mannitol	soy oil	whey
cottonseed oil	high fructose corn	methylcellulose	soy protein	whey powder
cyclodextrin	syrup (HFCS)	milk powder	soy protein isolate	xanthan gum

Visit: www.nongmoshoppingguide.com/ to download the above list of GM foods
Visit: www.responsibletechnology.org
Visit: www.greenerchoices.org/eco-labels/to learn about organic labels

Say No to MSG

MSG is a food additive that enhances flavors in food. It helps replace flavor lost by elimination of fat in many low-fat and no-fat foods which are so popular today. Monosodium glutamate was invented in 1908 in Japan. Use of the product was minimal in our country until after World War II, when it was introduced to the US food industry as a flavoring agent that our military discovered made Japanese army rations more palatable than our own. Shortly after MSG appeared in groceries stories in a product called "Accent." The debate over the safety of MSG goes back to 1968, when a Chinese physician wrote a letter titled "Chinese Restaurant Syndrome", to *The New England Journal of Medicine* [2] to ask for help in determining why he and his friends suffered numbness, weakness, and palpitations when they dined in certain Chinese restaurants. About the same time, John W. Olney, M.D., a neuroscientist at Washington University ran numerous studies on mice being fed MSG. He concluded that glutamic acid is a neurotoxin that kills brain neurons. Dr. Russell Blaylock, a board-certified neurosurgeon and author of "*Excitotoxins: The Taste that Kills*" explains that MSG is an excitotoxin, which means it overexcites your cells to the point of damage or death, causing brain damage to varying degrees -- and potentially even triggering or worsening learning disabilities, Alzheimer's disease, Parkinson's disease, Lou Gehrig's disease and more.[3]

The flavor and health benefits of real foods are far superior to processed, MSG-laden foods.

When food shopping please read your labels. Here's what to look out for:

These ALWAYS contain MSG:

Autolyzed yeast	Hydrolyzed corn gluten	Natrium glutamate	Yeast extracts
Calcium caseinate	Hydrolyzed protein	*(natrium in Latin/*	Yeast food
Gelatin	Monosodium glutamate	*German for sodium*	Yeast nutrient
Glutamate	Monopotassium	Sodium caseinate	
Glutamic acid	glutamate	Textured protein	

These often contain MSG or create MSG during processing:

Barley malt	Malt flavoring	Protease	Soy sauce extract
Bouillon and Broth	Maltodextrin	Protease enzymes	Stock
Carrageenan	Natural beef flavoring	Protein fortified	Ultra-pasteurized
Citric acid	Natural chicken	Seasonings	Whey protein
Enzymes	flavoring	Soy protein	Whey protein
Enzyme modified	Natural flavor &	Soy protein concentrate	concentrate
Anything fermented	flavorings	Soy protein isolate	Whey protein isolate
Flavors & flavorings	Natural pork flavoring	Soy sauce	
Malt extract	Pectin		

Visit: tv.naturalnews.com/ for more information on MSG
Visit: www.truthinlabeling.com for more information on food additives.

---

[2] www.price-pottenger.org, see MSG Dangers and Deceptions by Jack L. Samuels, Journal Issue: Vo l22, No 2
* Become a member and join to access this article as well as thousands of relating articles on health and nutrition
[3] Mercola, Joseph, articles.mercola.com/

References

Books

Carper, Jean. The Food Pharmacy, Bantam Books, N.Y., 1988
Chopra, Deepak. The Spontaneous Fulfillment of Desire, 2003
Colbin, Annemarie. The Natural Gourmet, Bantam Books, N.Y., 1989
David, Mark. Nourishing Wisdom, Bell Tower N.Y., 1991
Erasmus, Udo. Fats that Heal, Fats that Kill, ALIVE Books, Canada, 1986
Fuhrman, Joel, M.D., Eat for Health; Andi Score, Gift of Health Press, 2008
Gittleman, Ann Louise, M.S., C.N.S. Fat Flush Plan, McGraw-Hill N.Y.2002
Hadady, Letha, D.A.C. Asian Health Secrets, Three River Press, N.Y. 1996
Hippocrates Health Institute, Drs. Anna Maria and Brian Clement, West Palm Beach, Fl
Ignarro, Louis J.,M.D. No More Heart Disease, St. Martin's Press, N.Y.2005
Kushi, Michio. The Book of Macrobiotics, Tokyo Japan Publications 1977
Kushi, Michio.The Macrobiotic Way, Penguin Group, N.Y., 1985
London, Sheryl and Mel. The Versatile Grain & Elegant Bean, Simon and Schuster 1992
Long, Ruthanne and Dixon. Markets of Provence, Collins Publishers, Ca. 1996
Oshsawa, George. Zen Macrobiotics, Revised by Lou Oles, L.A., 1965
Pitchford Paul. Healing with Whole Foods, North Atlantic Books, Berkeley, Ca. 1993
Roizen, Michael, M.D. Puma, John, M.D., Cooking the Realage Way, Harper Collins, N.Y. 2003
Rose, Natalia, The Raw Food Detox Diet, HarperCollins Publishers, N.Y. 2005
Spector Platt, Ellen. Garlic, Onion & other Alliums, Stackpole Books, Pa. 2003
Thacker, Emily. The Vinegar Book, Tresco, Ohio 1995

Websites

Weil, Andrew, M.D., Daley, Rosie. The Healthy Kitchen, Alfred A. Knopt, N.Y. 2002
Werle, Loukie. Italian Country Cooking, Metro Books, N.Y., 2007
Williams, Roger. Nutrition Against Disease, Health is Wealth, Ca. 1962
Wong, Kumfoo. Sushi Made Easy, Sterling Publishers Co., N.Y., 1999
Wood, Rebecca. The Splendid Grain, William Morrow and Co., N.Y. 1997

Publications

Alternatives, Dr. David Williams; www.drdavidwilliams.com
Hippocrates Health Institute, Drs. Anna Maria and Brian Clement, West Palm Beach, Fl
Natural News. Mike Adams, Editor. The Health Ranger; www.naturalnews.com
Price-Pottenger Nutrition Foundation; www.ppnf.org
Weston A. Price Foundation; www.westonaprice.com

Informative Websites to Visit

www.cornucopia.org
www.eco-labels.org
www.ewg.org
www.greenerchoices.com
www.Hippocratesinstitute.org
www.localharvest.org
www.organic.org

References from the Introduction

1. According to the Cornucopia Institute even organic 70% organic products may contain some Hexane. To learn about the use of hexane in the health industry- and in soy products in particular- go to the Cornucopia Institute http://www.cornucopia.org/2010/11/hexane-soy/

2. USDA figures on GMO soy: www.ers.usda.gov/

3. For the most comprehensive information on this subject go to the Price-Pottenger Nutrition Foundation *(PPNF)* ppnf.org/ also known as the Health and Healing Wisdom Foundation. This is one of my favorite resources. It is a nonprofit public benefit corporation organized in 1965 as a nutrition education foundation. I use their valuable information on nutrition, diet and health in all of my teaching workshops.

4. Today, just navigating through the market place is a humble necessity almost like an art form. My website has a great free hand-out called, "Ten Manageable Tips for Shopping the Markets". I encourage you to print it out and use it.

5. Dirty Dozen and Clean 15 : www.ewg.org/

6. You can join the team by mailing a check to: Carol Blumenfeld's office/ MSKCC, 633 3rd Avenue, 28th floor, New York, New York 10017. (Checks made payable to MSKCC, kindly write on the memo: For the "Whit Whit Fund".)

Acknowledgments

This book has become a real family effort, for this I appreciate and thank my family all.

First, I thank my son Christian for pulling together the manuscript for the final steps of the book. His organizational skills are one of his many talents. His patience and kindness is a blessing in my life.

To my sister JoAnna for stepping in and making my introduction come alive. She has been a wonderful mentor to me during this project. With her experience as a great writer and editor and knowledge of healthy, delicious food she gave inspiring suggestions that enriched these pages.

My deepest gratitude to my husband Anthony for being a sounding board for ideas that began years ago. His creative touch to everything has helped me greatly pull together beautiful pictures and ideas and some creative copy. A special thanks to him for tasting all my crazy creations over the years and putting up with much chaos in the kitchen.

To my daughter Melina for helping with editing and her enlightening ideas and informative input. To my niece, photographer Jeanine Brandi McLychok for much editing and friendly - smart suggestions. Her many exquisite food pictures grace this book as well as my website.

Many special thanks to Kerin McElhenny for great editing. Many special thanks to my daughter-in-law Lela Bari for her talent as an editor, health counselor and true natural foodie and her special creative eye for staging some of the photos. To my food editor Heidi Fagley for her fantastic energy and expertise as a Chef and editor on checking every recipe for perfection.

My heartfelt thanks to Chef Jill Engelheart for her helping hand with the Asian section. Her skills as a Natural Chef and her generosity of spirit pulled that section together. Loving thanks to Beth V. Williams for her beautiful illustrations that reflect the special artist and loving mother she is, as well as an amazing soulful cook. My thanks to photographer Franziska S. Lewis. My special thanks to Jill Johnson for the wonderful photography. A big thank you to Tom Decker for his cover photography. Thanks to the team at Good Pep Designs for creating and managing social media for this book. Thanks to the Balboa Press publication team for their endless coaching and support.

To all my sister friends for standing by me for years assisting me in cooking, and trying out all my intensely healthy crazy creations. They are: Karen DeLuca, Patti Taylor, Celia Goodstein, Jessica Starke, Christine Lupo, Margaret and Katie Corrado, and Fran Sadis. I thank them always for their nurturing support and believing in me. A special thanks to Chrissey Calamari for her talents in assisting with the cover photo. For many loyal customers especially; Stacey Satovsky, Sarah Goldblatt, Tracy Possicillo, for giving me advice, positive feedback and encouraging me to be a better Chef than I am.

And finally I want to express my love and gratitude to Dr. Annemarie Colbin for starting a humble cooking school in her apartment which led to the founding of "The Natural Gourmet Institute for Health & Culinary Arts" in 1977. They are now the leader in teaching health-supportive cooking as well as elucidating the relationship between food and health. Attending her school in the beginning of the nineties forever changed my life.

Working on this book was a special joy for me. I am honored and grateful to be in this profession. I know I am where I am supposed to be.

Index

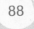

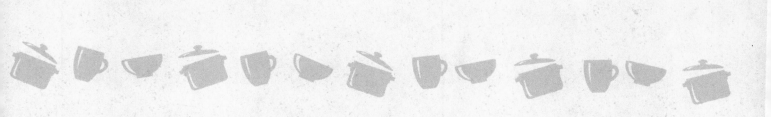

CPSIA information can be obtained
at www.ICGtesting.com
Printed in the USA
JSHW061126080223
37406JS00001B/1